ALZHEIMER'S

Caring for Your Loved One

Caring for Yourself

Sharon Fish

with Susan Cuthbert

A LION BOOK

First published in Great Britain in 1991 by
Lion Publishing plc
Sandy Lane West, Oxford, England

This edition first published in 1997

A catalogue record of this book is available from the British Library
ISBN 0 7459 3442 0

Albatross Books Pty Ltd
P O Box 320, Sutherland, NSW 2232, Australia
ISBN 0 7324 1447 4

Adapted for the United Kingdom by Susan Cuthbert
Printed and bound in the United Kingdom by Cox & Wyman

Acknowledgments

My hope for all who read this book is that you will be encouraged. You are not alone as you reach out to care for your loved ones and as you are cared for yourself.

I am deeply grateful to Jack Fisher, Kathleen Fisher Poling, Marian Gierasch and Mary Butts, four caregivers who formed the Alzheimer's support group in Oneonta, New York, and who have faithfully kept the candle burning for nearly a decade for those who need to know they're not alone.

Special thanks to Mary Johnson, who read the manuscript, and to the dozens of other caregivers who were willing to share their experiences for others to learn from, including me. To protect caregivers' privacy, no names are included and, in some instances, certain identifying details have been changed at their request. Scenarios that introduce various chapters weave together all our stories, our fears, our hopes, our feelings. The people described could well be your mother or father, husband or wife, sister or brother, son or daughter.

I would like to thank Dr. Raymond Vickers, MD, medical director of the New York State Veterans' Home, Oxford, New York, who read and edited the manuscript with a doctor's eye; and also his wife, Barbara, who gives so generously of her time and talents to encourage caregivers throughout our region.

Thank you to the following people who have lovingly cared for my mother in our home or theirs over the past ten years: Sylvia Davisson, Pat Gifford, Janet Roseboom, Bunny Rodriquez, Kim Lund, Carol Rose, Katie Jenison, and Debbie Derry. Thanks to the staff at Stamford Nursing Home in Stamford, New York, who cared for my mother as if she were *their* mother during the final days of her life. And thank you to the staff and friends of Inter County Home Care, who have always been there when I needed them.

Special thanks to the following for a number of reasons: Peg and Frank MacCracken and Norman Moran, who offered wisdom and support; Dr Steven Szebenyi and Dr Donald Pollock from Bassett Hospital, Coopertown, New York, who have helped me over the years with medical management; Helen and David Moberg, two people who have built into my life over the miles; Granger Westberg, whose commitment to holistic health has challenged me to a more balanced lifestyle; and the editors of *The Freeman's Journal*, Cooperstown, New York, who first published my caregiving column that eventually grew into book proportions.

My final thanks go to Hazel (Grandma) Brown, who prayed; to friends and relatives who encouraged; and to my mother, Pearle Fish, who was always a caregiver and who was always loving.

I am grateful.

Sharon Fish

Acknowledgments from the UK editor

With grateful thanks to Clive Evers for the benefit of his special knowledge. Also to Mrs Joan King and the Oxfordshire Branch of the Alzheimer's Disease Society, to my friends Janet Hathaway, Mari-an Watkins, Janet Baraclough, Sarah Moore, Bridget Banks and Dr Peter Garside, and to my mother-in-law Mrs Hazel Cuthbert, for their help with the finer details of the 'Anglicization'. It has been much appreciated, though of course responsibility for any deficiencies rests firmly with me.

Susan Cuthbert

CONTENTS

Part One

SOMETHING HAS GONE WRONG

*A bruised reed he will not break,
and a dimly burning wick he will not
quench.*
THE BOOK OF ISAIAH

CHAPTER ONE

Bruised Reeds and Dimly Burning Wicks

Muriel sat down at the kitchen table and slowly buttered her toast. Fifteen minutes of silence, twenty if she was lucky. Quiet time alone to enjoy the toast, a cup of coffee, and a quick read through the morning paper before the real work began: getting her mother up, washed, fed, toileted, walked, and dressed for the day. And then, later in the morning, several loads of laundry including her mother's urine-stained sheets.

'Bye, Mum,' Susan shouted as she grabbed her books and headed out of the door to catch the school bus.

'Bye,' yelled Bruce, scooping up his rucksack and racing past his sister.

Muriel glanced out the window and caught a glimpse of the bus as it rounded the curve and disappeared out of sight beyond the hedgerow.

The school term would be over in a few weeks. Unfortunately, Muriel knew the children weren't looking forward to being home all summer. When she'd asked them they said they didn't mind, but her neighbour had told her the truth. When the neighbour had asked Susan how she was going to spend her summer holiday, Susan had just shrugged her

13

shoulders and looked unhappy. And Bruce said, 'We aren't going anywhere because of Grandma.'

'Mur. Mur.'

'Ten of my twenty minutes wasted thinking about something I can't do anything about,' Muriel thought.

'Mur. Mur.'

'In a minute, Mother,' Muriel called back, hastily swallowing the last of the coffee, running her plate under the tap and shoving it into the dishwasher.

Ruth. Muriel's mother. Ruth was the reason the children weren't looking forward to their summer holiday.

Muriel couldn't blame them. It wasn't easy being thirteen and seven and having a grandparent with Alzheimer's disease living with you twenty-four hours a day. A grandmother who didn't do the things grandmothers were supposed to do—like tell you what clever grandchildren you were, listen to your stories and bake you biscuits. A grandmother who, instead, sometimes threatened you and didn't even know your name, babbled incoherently at times, and had almost burned your house down trying to boil an egg.

Muriel's father had died fifteen years earlier, and her mother never remarried. Ruth continued to live alone in the old family farmhouse, three miles from Muriel, Carl and the children. At age sixty-five, Ruth had begun to show signs of memory loss, but the signs were so subtle that Muriel hardly noticed them.

Her mother was for ever losing things: her glasses, her cheque-book, her keys. When Muriel would drop in unexpectedly she'd often find Ruth rummaging through drawers, muttering under her breath. But then, for as long as Muriel could remember, her mother had misplaced things.

Then her mother stopped remembering.

Birthdays were first. Muriel's. Carl's. Susan's. Bruce's.

14

Her own. Very unlike the mother who had never failed to send a card, buy a present or bake a cake.

Appointments were next. The dentist, hairdresser, chiropodist—all were forgotten. Muriel had phone calls from all three of them one month asking where Ruth was.

Muriel's mother had notes posted all over the house. 'Memory joggers,' Ruth called them. But she still forgot.

And then there were names. Odd, Muriel had thought, that her mother couldn't seem to remember the names of the children one Sunday when she was over for dinner. Ruth kept calling them Sally and Ron, the names of her own sister and brother. The children thought it was a game Grandma was playing. Muriel wasn't so sure.

It was Muriel's husband, Carl, who first realized there was more wrong with Ruth than simple age-related memory loss.

Carl stopped by the farm one morning to get Ruth's shopping list and found his mother-in-law taking a nap in a smoke-filled house. She had put a fruit cake in the oven, turned the oven on high and gone to sleep. The smoke detector was working, but Ruth had removed her hearing aid and, as she told them later, had forgotten where she put it. A look in the kitchen cupboards revealed more black-bottomed cake tins and saucepans, ample evidence that cooking was one task Ruth could no longer accomplish safely.

The final straw came several weeks later when Muriel got a phone call. Ruth was at the post office in town, having walked the two miles in the rain. She insisted she was in the bank, wanted to see the balance on her account, and demanded her money. Could Muriel please come and get her mother, asked the postmistress.

Muriel did. She got Ruth, took her home to the farm and started packing.

Moving hadn't been easy. Ruth became even more con-

15

fused and disorientated in the new environment. She accused Muriel and Carl of stealing her money and selling the family farm.

The children, then aged ten and four, were a mixed blessing as far as Ruth was concerned. Sometimes she showered them with affection, and they basked in the attention. At other times they were also part of the supposed conspiracy to confiscate her property.

Bruce seemed to go with the flow of Grandma's mood swings, but Susan, who had known the love of a more stable grandmother, had a difficult time accepting the bizarre behaviour patterns that emerged. When Ruth had one of her verbal outbursts, Susan would run to her own room and stay there until her mother or father assured her the coast was clear.

Now, three years later, Ruth's paranoia was gone, but Susan's habit of retreat remained. Muriel hoped Susan would outgrow it. And she wished she didn't feel so guilty about the children.

'Mur. Mur,' Ruth called from the bedroom, the room Susan had given up when her grandmother moved in.

'Coming, Mother,' Muriel called, as she dried her hands on the tea towel and turned to go upstairs.

Alzheimer's: A Family Affair

This book is certainly not the first word on Alzheimer's disease, nor will it be the last. Rather it is one voice in a chorus speaking out about a devastating illness affecting the daily lives of millions of people worldwide. People like Muriel and Ruth. People like my mother and your mother, our fathers, husbands, wives, children. The cared for and the carers. The loved ones and those who love.

I am a carer and writer as well as a registered nurse. Twenty years of hospital, nursing-home and home-nursing experience have brought me in contact with many carers and their loved ones. But my own mother brought the reality of Alzheimer's home. In 1980 she was diagnosed with senile dementia of the Alzheimer's type, and I was able to experience caregiving firsthand for over ten years, from the time I first moved home to help my father cope until her death in a nursing home. In 1989 I decided it was time to write about the things my mother taught me and the things I've learned from other carers.

The scenarios that introduce various chapters in this book are based on the lives of many carers including myself. In them, I've tried to weave together our experiences, reminiscences and feelings to paint a picture of what Alzheimer's is really like.

This book is primarily for carers like myself—those who live with loved ones, visit them in nursing homes and sheltered homes, or show care and concern from afar. I also hope it will be of value to professional and voluntary carers who recognize illness as a family affair. And, too, I wrote it for friends. Without them, caring would be a very lonely experience.

In addition to drawing from my own experience and current research and literature, I interviewed dozens of carers who gave me permission to quote them. This gave direction for chapter topics and helped me focus on some primary concerns. The inclusion of appendices in this edition was designed with the professional caregiver in mind and for family caregivers needing additional sources of information.

Whenever people talk about Alzheimer's, certain questions come up.

● How can I tell if my loved one has Alzheimer's? What are the early signs and symptoms?

- What causes Alzheimer's disease? Is it hereditary?

- How can I be sure my friend or relative is getting an accurate diagnosis? What's involved in the diagnostic process?

- What are some of the bizarre and bewildering behaviours peculiar to Alzheimer's disease? How can I manage them?

- Is there any specific treatment or cure?

- What's the purpose for all this suffering? Why should God allow this to happen?

- How can I meet my own needs as a wife, husband, daughter, son?

- Is it normal for me to feel angry, guilty, depressed and resentful? How can I deal with these emotions?

- How can I deal with my loved one's physical needs?

- What kinds of resources are available to help care for an Alzheimer's sufferer at home? How can I find and pay for this care?

- How can a person decide to place a relative in a nursing home? Is there ever a right time?

- Are brain post-mortems important? How can I find out about them?

- What will death be like for my loved one? What will his or her death be like for me?

We will look at each of these questions in detail in later chapters. But first, what is Alzheimer's? Who gets it?

Some Facts about Alzheimer's

Alzheimer's disease is a chronic, progressive, irreversible brain disorder or dementia for which there is no definable cause, no definitive treatment and, to date, no foreseeable cure.

Dementia is a multifaceted decline of intellectual functions of sufficient severity to interfere with an individual's activities of daily living, career, social relationships and social activities. Dementia involves personality changes, loss of memory and judgement, and difficulty with abstract thinking and orientation.

The word *dementia* literally means 'mind away' or 'deprived of mind.' Dementing illnesses are the result of one or more disease processes that can drastically alter people's behaviour and gradually bankrupt their minds and the lives of entire families. Alzheimer's disease is thought to be the primary cause of incurable dementia for men and women over the age of sixty-five.

In Britain there are about seven and a half million people over sixty-five years of age. Of this population, more than 750,000 people may suffer from Alzheimer's disease. Statistics are similar in other developed countries where life expectancy reaches into the sixties and seventies.

Although Alzheimer's usually occurs after a person reaches the mid-sixties, with a significant increase after age eighty, Alzheimer's can also afflict people in their forties and fifties. It's not just a disease of the old or very old.

By the turn of the century, the numbers of people suffering from dementia in Britain alone will be over one million. The accompanying emotional and economic costs stagger the imagination. While the majority of people with Alzheimer's continue to live in a home environment supported by friends, relatives and community services, it is estimated that Alzheimer's sufferers currently fill about 60 per cent of all nursing-home beds.

A leading cause of death in people older than seventy-five, Alzheimer's has been called 'the disease of the twentieth century.' It may well be the disease of the twenty-first century as well: as the over eighty-five population doubles, one out of every three of us may have an older relative diagnosed with Alzheimer's.

Alzheimer's disease has also been described as 'a funeral that never ends,' 'a nightmare from which you never wake up,' 'another name for madness,' 'the silent epidemic,' 'the slow death of the mind.' One of the most popular and practical books ever written on the subject of Alzheimer's disease is titled *The 36-Hour Day*, reflecting the reality of life for most carers.

Caring for a loved one with a dementing illness does seem to require more than seven days a week, twenty-four hours a day, sixty minutes an hour; the difficulties inherent in caring for someone with Alzheimer's disease are only too real.

But the difficulties are not the whole picture. Caring can also be an opportunity for growth. It can make us more patient, more compassionate and more courageous people.

A beautiful passage in the Bible reads, 'A bruised reed he will not break, and a dimly burning wick he will not quench.' There is hope for the carer who feels battered and bruised in the battle against Alzheimer's disease. We need not be broken.

There is also hope for our loved ones. No matter how bizarre or bewildering their behaviour, they are still precious people carefully designed in the likeness of their creator. As carers we have daily opportunities to fan the flames of their hearts and spirits as we care for them in love.

And, it is hoped, our own hearts and spirits will be lifted

up and comforted in the very process of caring as we discover untapped, unrecognized strengths in ourselves and in the people around us.

CHAPTER TWO

Searching for the Truth

'I think my mother has Alzheimer's,' a friend confided to me over the phone one night. 'She has all the symptoms your mother does. She's confused and forgetful. She can't even remember her own name or mine, and she's having a lot of personality changes.'

'How long has this been going on?' I asked, puzzled because this was the first time my friend had mentioned her mother's changing behaviour.

'Just about a month,' she said.

I told my friend her mother's condition might not be the more gradually developing disease of Alzheimer's and encouraged her to take her mother to a doctor immediately.

My friend's mother was diagnosed a short time later. She didn't have Alzheimer's. She had a rapidly growing brain tumour.

In past decades, Alzheimer's was one of the most under-diagnosed diseases. Today it has burst out of obscurity to become one of the most overdiagnosed, particularly among friends and family members who have read a lot about it in the popular literature.

Even some health-care professionals are guilty of making the instant diagnosis. Unfortunately, it's still not uncommon to hear people say, 'My husband's doctor took one look at him and said, "He has all the symptoms of Alzheimer's. It's not necessary to run any tests."'

Yet brain post-mortem reports have indicated that a significant number of people actually diagnosed with Alzheimer's did not in fact have Alzheimer's. They showed none of Alzheimer's characteristic physical changes in the brain, even though they had exhibited symptoms of brain dementia. (Characteristic physical changes include senile plaques and neurofibrillary tangles that form in the brain tissue of people with Alzheimer's.)

Alzheimer's is not the *only* disease process that causes dementia. Far from it. There are more than fifty different disorders whose symptoms can mimic those of Alzheimer's disease. While some of these disorders are chronic and incurable, many others can be treated, reversed or cured completely. Many have nothing to do with the brain at all in relation to cause. Some of theses disorders may also coexist with Alzheimer's, exaggerating symptoms.

There is always the need, in the case of memory loss and confusion, to have a complete diagnostic examination as soon as possible. This is true whether the confusion is mild or severe, whatever the person's age. The examination should include a thorough history and check-up, various blood tests, a neurological and psychological assessment and, in some cases, a psychiatric evaluation.

Diagnosing Alzheimer's is a laborious process of elimination and exclusion. One visit to the doctor will not usually result in a diagnosis. Nor will one test.

Never feel guilty about seeking a second opinion. Diagnosis is difficult. The course of the disease process varies greatly from person to person, and there is always a degree of diagnostic uncertainty.

Members of Alzheimer's support groups can be particularly helpful in steering you to sensitive doctors. You'll want a GP you can talk to and trust because you'll probably be seeing a lot of each other. You will also appreciate one who is prepared to make home visits when necessary.

If you wish to change your GP, you may ask the current doctor to sign your relative's card and take this to the new doctor. Alternatively you may send the medical card directly to the local Family Practitioner Committee (F.P.C.) stating your relative's wish to change doctors. Evaluating a person for Alzheimer's is not a once-in-a-lifetime experience. Certain tests may need to be repeated at yearly or more frequent intervals as the disease progresses, especially with the younger Alzheimer's sufferer. Early symptoms of Alzheimer's disease are subtle, but if your relative has Alzheimer's there will be a definite downhill progression. People with Alzheimer's do not get better.

For your own peace of mind and for the health of your loved one, never assume it's Alzheimer's until all the test results are in.

Historical Highlights

> Actually, when we think back, Dad started to act depressed after his colostomy surgery in 1968. He felt he was not normal. But then there was more than just the depression. From that point on it seemed all downhill. There were other signs. He was about sixty-four.

As carers, *we ourselves* are the single most important diagnostic tool in the search for truth about what's causing our loved one's confusion. Our reflections on the history of his or her behaviour changes are invaluable to the doctor. Though most doctors will want to question a patient directly, people in the early stages of Alzheimer's can be masters in the fine art of 'cover-up.' Not a few doctors have been fooled by the perfectly normal behaviour and appearance of people with Alzheimer's in their surgery. You know things are different at home, but you may need some facts to prove it.

When attempting to reconstruct a medical and social history, there are two key words to remember: *change* and *onset*.

What are the various changes you've noticed in your loved one's life over the past few weeks, months or years? When did you first notice these changes? Have they been gradual in onset, occurring over a period of time, or have they occurred suddenly?

The time frame for the appearance and progression of symptoms is an important clue for doctors to consider when making a diagnosis and deciding what tests to conduct. Before you go to the hospital or the GP's surgery, think through the following categories. You may even want to write down your answers and take them with you.

Circumstances and attitudes. Has your loved one been unusually anxious, agitated, depressed, apathetic or withdrawn? When did you first notice these changes? Have there been any major events associated with these changes, such as retirement, relocation, death of a close friend or relative, surgery?

Behaviour. What specific behaviour changes have you noticed? Have there been any differences in your loved one's daily routine? Have you noticed any marked personality changes, such as forgetfulness? If so, what exactly is forgotten?

Conversation. Has your loved one experienced any language difficulties? Have there been any problems related to the ability to speak or remember words? Is one word substituted for another at the end of a sentence? Are phrases mixed up or confused? Has speech become slurred or garbled?

Decision making. Have you noticed any changes in decision-making capabilities? Are there any errors in judgement? In relation to what, specifically? Is your loved one having difficulty driving? Has he or she ever wandered off and got lost?

Drugs. List any medications being taken, both prescription and over-the-counter. Are medications being taken correctly?

Environment. Are saucepans burned? Are there piles of unpaid bills? Is post stacked up? Is there evidence that your relative is neglecting nutritional needs?

Family and friends. What have other people—friends, neighbours, co-workers—noticed in relation to your loved one's behaviour?

Grooming and gait disturbances. Is there any change in the person's ability to perform various activities of daily living related to personal grooming—bathing, dressing, toileting? Have there been any changes in the ability to walk?

Habits. What changes have you noticed in your loved one's normal habit patterns? Are there things that are simply too difficult to do now, such as balancing a cheque-book, cooking, cleaning, reading, car repair, gardening? Are there any favourite hobbies that are no longer engaged in? Have you noticed any changes in the ability and desire to socialize with others?

Illnesses. What specific physical symptoms is your loved one experiencing? Has there been any weight loss or gain?

Is there a history of any of the following: metabolic disorders such as diabetes or thyroid disease, heart or lung abnormalities, strokes, dizziness, fainting spells, headaches, shaking, seizures? Is there any history of alcoholism?

Has your loved one fallen down or had any past or recent head injuries? Has there been exposure to any toxic chemicals in the work place? Is there any history of blood transfusions? When and where were they done? Is there any history of Alzheimer's disease or undiagnosed memory loss in your loved one's family? Any familial nervous or mental disease?

As carers we need to be sure that no stone has been left unturned in the search for the cause of our loved one's confusion. The stones related to our loved one's history are the ones we need to turn over ourselves.

Maybe It's Not Alzheimer's

In the beginning we said to ourselves, 'Dad is just getting old.' Even his doctor said so and told us it was probably just hardening of the arteries to the brain. So we thought, well, he's getting old and he's getting senile.

But his confusion wasn't just part of old age, we found out later. We finally took him to a doctor who listened to him, did a good examination, a bunch of tests, and was willing to tell us more about what was going on.

A good place to start in the search for truth about the cause of our loved one's confusion is with a general physical examination. This will involve more than taking a temperature, pulse and blood pressure.

Even if the primary dementia is caused by Alzheimer's, there may be associated chronic or acute problems. If these go undiagnosed and untreated, they can make the confusion caused by Alzheimer's worse. On the other hand, some of these conditions may themselves be the cause of the confusion.

Chronic and acute diseases and disabilities. Heart or lung related diseases such as congestive heart failure, heart-rhythm and valve disorders, pneumonia and a variety of chronic obstructive lung disorders may contribute to mild or severe oxygen deprivation to the brain. This lack of oxygen, in turn, can cause acute episodes of confusion and can contribute to chronic dementia.

In some cases the culprit of confusion is a chronic atherana build-up that results in a narrowing of the arteries supplying blood to the brain. This is called coronary artery disease or atherosclerosis. Coronary artery disease (usually with accompanying hypertension) may, over a period of time, result in a series of small strokes or infarcts in the brain. This can cause an intermittent confusion that is frequently mistaken for Alzheimer's disease and often goes undetected unless the person experiences a massive stroke.

This mini-stroke phenomenon, more frequently seen in men, is called multi-infarct dementia or vascular dementia. It is the second most common cause of confusion in older people, responsible for approximately thirty-five per cent of all dementias.

Unlike Alzheimer's, multi-infarct dementia often begins suddenly. Its downhill progression is usually steplike in nature, with plateaus. There may be evidence of specific local or focal neurological impairments such as muscle weakness to an arm or leg or slurred speech, as opposed to the more gradual and generalized global decline of Alzheimer's disease. By supplying the person's history, a carer may help the doctor distinguish between Alzheimer's and multi-infarct dementia.

People can, and frequently do, suffer from multi-infarct dementia in combination with Alzheimer's. Why is it important to know which problem is causing the person's confusion? Medical and/or surgical treatments can often eliminate or greatly reduce the likelihood of further stroke activity if the confusion is related to vascular disease rather than the Alzheimer's process. An accurate diagnosis can lead to improved health.

There are also other diseases that may produce progressive dementialike symptoms. The most notable are Huntington's chorea, Pick's disease, multiple sclerosis, amyotrophic lateral sclerosis, Parkinson's disease and Creutzfeldt-Jakob disease, an extremely rare brain disorder. An overview of these conditions is included in Appendix B.

Sensory impairments or disabilities may also be a factor in confusion. Occasionally when older people appear to be forgetful or confused they are simply suffering from poor vision and/or hearing loss. Both conditions may be correctable with surgery or mechanical aids.

Deficiencies. The brain needs nutritious food to survive. If it isn't adequately nourished it can become confused, forgetful, irritable and depressed.

People—especially older people who live alone—can suffer from a number of conditions that are diet related. If older people forget to eat, or fail to eat enough of the right kinds of foods, they may wind up with nutritional deficiencies and even chronic malnutrition. Chronic alcoholism can also be a concern. Both conditions are associated with vitamin deficiencies, and some vitamin deficiencies contribute to dementia like symptoms. If an older person is not drinking enough water, dehydration can also rapidly occur and contribute to lethargy and confusion and sometimes hallucinations. Food sensitivity can lead to confusion too.

Depression. Depression and manic depression are two other conditions that can mimic Alzheimer's and should always be considered when there is memory loss.

Classically depressed people may appear passive, helpless, hopeless and confused. Behavioural and intellectual responses may be slower than normal. Manic depression may result in mood changes that swing between a state of excitement, or mania, and deep depression.

The onset of depression is usually more rapid than the onset of Alzheimer's and may be triggered by specific events such as the death of a spouse or the loss of a job. There are often accompanying physical signs such as fatigue, insomnia, and loss of weight and appetite.

Twenty to twenty-five per cent of the time, depression accompanies Alzheimer's, thus exaggerating the symptoms of dementia. Although Alzheimer's cannot be cured, depression will often respond to anti-depressant medication.

Drugs. One of the most commonly overlooked yet correctable causes of confusion in older people is drug toxicity. The effects of many medications extend far beyond the therapeutic purposes for which they were intended. Many have potentially harmful side effects that can include depression, disorientation and other dementia-like symptoms.

Drug toxicity can result from either a build-up of one specific medication or a combination of drugs that can produce toxic effects, usually over time. It's not unusual for an older person to be taking a number of different medications, which they may have stored up over a long period. Some of these drugs can neutralize other drugs when taken together. Or they can do the exact opposite and speed up the absorption of the second drug, often to an overdose level. All drugs, including those we may think of as innocuous over-the-counter pain relievers, cough suppressants and laxatives, have potential side effects.

Medications have a greater tendency to build up in the bodies of older people because of the decreased filtration rate in the kidneys. Poor circulation, slower general metabolism, constipation and a lower level of liver detoxification function contribute to drug toxicity as we age.

Medications can also adversely affect the proper absorption of vitamins, minerals and other nutrients. Overuse of some antacids, for example, can trigger thiamine deficiencies. Medications can also contribute to nutritional and electrolyte imbalances that, in turn, can create confusion. Even something as ordinary as a laxative, if taken indiscriminately, can upset fluid and electrolyte balances.

Older people sometimes consume alcohol in the form of wine or over-the-counter cough medicines or liquid vitamin supplements. Alcohol does not mix well with many medications. Confusion is a common side effect.

When we take our loved one to the hospital or doctor's surgery we need to take their medications too, both prescription and over-the-counter, or at least have an accurate record of what they are taking and how long they've been taking it. Medication should definitely be considered as a contributing factor whenever dementia is suspected.

Lab Tests Don't Lie

I think they did every test imaginable on my husband to make sure he wasn't suffering from something other than Alzheimer's. At forty-five, you want to make sure.

No examination for Alzheimer's would be complete without blood analysis and other laboratory tests. All of them

31

help to rule out other possible causes of dementia. While not every test will be used by every doctor on every person showing symptoms of dementia, some of these certainly will be performed.

Blood tests. A full blood count (FBC) should be done to rule out the possibility of any underlying acute or chronic infectious process that can cause symptoms similar to Alzheimer's. The FBC can also detect other conditions such as blood cancers or anaemia. Low haemoglobin and haematocrit levels can contribute to confusion when there are not enough red blood cells carrying oxygen to the brain.

More specific blood chemistries can measure folic acid and vitamin B12 levels. Low vitamin B12 levels may be associated with pernicious anaemia. Symptoms are depression and irritability. Low B12 and folate levels also produce dementia-like symptoms.

Diabetes and other metabolic or endocrine disorders can contribute to marked irritability, personality changes and confusion. They can be detected by blood tests.

Abnormally high or low doses of thyroid hormone can trigger dementia-like symptoms and can be detected through various thyroid hormone level studies. Abnormally high levels of circulating calcium and sodium and low sodium levels with accompanying electrolyte imbalances can also trigger symptoms of dementia.

Poisoning with certain metals such as aluminium, manganese, lead or mercury has been implicated in dementia as have pesticides, carbon monoxide and industrial pollutants. Blood levels can be tested for many of these.

In the nineteenth century, the number-one cause of confusion was thought to be syphilis. While it is not generally a major cause of dementia today, a complete assessment for dementia should include a blood test for chronic venereal disease.

Acquired immune deficiency syndrome (AIDS) is another infectious process that can't be automatically ruled out. Dementia is a frequent complication of AIDS. Blood studies to detect the presence of the AIDS virus may be done if the symptoms and health history indicate a need.

Urine tests. Urine testing can rule out an acute urinary-tract infection that, in the elderly, may cause confusion. High sugar and acetone readings in the urine can also indicate diabetes and the need for more extensive blood work. Urine and blood tests may also reveal evidence of medication overdose.

Spinal fluid tests. The spinal column is part of the central nervous system. The cerebral spinal fluid courses through the spinal column also bathes the brain.

Spinal taps, or lumbar punctures (LPs), are recommended by some doctors as a diagnostic tool if there is a reason to suspect they would help rule out an infectious process. In this procedure, a small amount of spinal fluid is withdrawn from the spinal column, then analyzed.

Brain tumours, some blood-vessel diseases, and acute and chronic infectious processes such as meningitis and tuberculosis may be diagnosed through spinal taps.

The Mind Matters

When my mother was initially diagnosed with senile dementia of the Alzheimer's type, I went into the examining room with her when she saw the neurologist. I can still remember the 'conversation' my mother had with the young neurology resident.

'I just want to ask you a few questions,' the resident began.

'Okay,' my mother replied.

'What year is it?' he asked.

'1960,' she said.

'No, it's 1980,' he corrected her. 'What month is it?'

'May,' she said.

'No, it's December,' he said. 'What date is it now?'

'The first. Is that right?' my mother asked.

'No, it's the tenth,' he told her. 'What is the day of the week?'

'You're so clever, you tell me,' said Mum.

That concluded the mental-status exam.

What year is it now? What month is it? What date? What day of the week? For most of us, answers to these questions trip off our tongues without much thought. But for someone with a progressive memory loss like Alzheimer's, even the simplest questions can draw a blank.

> The doctor never actually saw my father's bizarre behaviour. He wondered if it was my mother's imagination. Until he could see the problems for himself, he wouldn't believe her.
>
> The doctor finally took Dad into a room and asked him some questions.
>
> Dad didn't know if he was married. He didn't know his religion. He didn't know who the prime minister was. He didn't know the month or the day or the season.
>
> The doctor finally realized my mother had been telling the truth.

A neurologist and/or the general practitioner may do a mental-status or mini-mental status exam. The various tests that are part of the exam indicate the ability of different parts of the brain to function. The more complex questions can give clues to the cause and progression of the dementia.

Mental-status exams generally measure what is known as

cognitive functioning. The word *cognition,* used extensively by health-care professionals when talking about the dementias, means 'the process or quality of knowing.' Cognition includes our ability to reason and remember, perceive and make judgements, conceive and imagine—all those mental activities that make us uniquely human, uniquely us.

Mental-status exams may be repeated over time to better assess our loved one's level of functioning and rate of change. The questions used test a number of different areas:

Degree of orientation to time, place, person. Do they know what day it is, where they are, who they are? Are they aware of current events? For example, do they know who the prime minister is? Do they know their phone number and their address? If shown familiar objects such as a pencil or a watch, can they name them?

Memory for remote and recent past. Can they tell when and where they were born? Do they know the names of their parents? Can they repeat from memory a simple series of numbers or familiar objects, five minutes after they are told what those numbers or objects are?

Mathematical skills. Can they solve simple maths calculations? For example, can they count backward from one hundred in multiples of three or four?

Abstract reasoning ability and judgement. Do they know the meaning of simple proverbs such as 'A bird in the hand is worth two in the bush'? If they were told that the cooker was on fire in their kitchen, what would they do? Is their response logical?

Reading, writing and symbolic drawing skills. Are they able to read? Do they understand what they are reading? Are they able to construct a sentence or a paragraph? Can they copy a simple design such as two overlapping triangles or rectangles? Can they draw the face of a clock and pencil-in the appropriate numbers in the right places?

We often take our minds for granted. The mental-status exam reminds us of how much they really do matter and of how they can be adversely affected by a disease such as Alzheimer's.

Having Your Head Examined

We're all familiar with the phrase, 'You ought to have your head examined.' This, in fact, may be just what the doctor orders for a confused person who might be suffering from Alzheimer's disease.

When my mother began having symptoms of memory loss, the last thing she wanted to do was to go to a doctor. 'I don't trust them,' she'd say when my father and I encouraged her to visit the nearby clinic.

I finally made an appointment with the practice nurse in our small town. I thought the fact that she was a woman might help make my mother feel more at ease, and I thought the small surgery would seem less imposing than a big hospital.

I was wrong on both counts.

My mother reluctantly agreed to the appointment, but we hadn't been in the waiting room more than five minutes when she headed out the door at top speed. 'I'm all right,' she insisted. 'All right.'

One day, after several more episodes like this, I got a phone call at work from the local supermarket. Mum had been in town making her usual morning rounds from post office to tea shop to supermarket. The manager had noticed my mother acting more confused than usual. 'The side of her mouth is drooping a bit,' he said. 'She's unsteady on her feet, but she keeps insisting she's okay and won't let me call an ambulance.'

I got in my car and drove the eight miles home in about five minutes. There was my mother coming out of the bank, leaning to the left. I knew the signs. She looked as if she'd had a small stroke.

'Get in the car, Mum,' I said.

'No.'

'Mum, please get in the car.'

'No,' she insisted.

Thankfully, my mother is small. I got out and manoeuvred her into the car, fastened her seat belt, and drove to the hospital. She protested all the way but calmed down as we neared the emergency entrance.

When we got there, I was able to speak to a doctor I knew. He seized the opportunity to admit her and then give her a brain or CAT scan. A short time later, she was officially diagnosed as having Alzheimer's. There was no evidence on the scan of any past stroke activity.

Other carers have shared their initial experiences with the diagnostic process:

> My wife had been going to one hospital for her eyes. Laser treatments. And one day her doctor said, 'You know, it wouldn't hurt your wife to have an MRI scan done.'
>
> I asked why.
>
> He said, 'Well, in talking to her there are times when she doesn't answer me.'
>
> I said to him, 'I know that. I thought she was just ignoring me.'
>
> 'No,' he said. 'It's much more than that.'

A thorough neurological examination for mental impairment may include an EEG, CAT or MRI scan either early in the investigative process or after more simple tests have been done without a diagnosis being made.

The *EEG* or electroencephalogram measures electrical activity in the brain. It involves attaching tiny wires called electrodes to the side of the head with a paste-like substance. The brain waves of people with Alzheimer's may appear perfectly normal, or they may show abnormally slow electrical activity.

EEGs can help identify other causes of dementia with symptoms that mimic Alzheimer's, such as delirium and various seizure disorders that may have gone undiagnosed or been misdiagnosed in the past.

A *CAT* scan, or a computerized axial tomogram, is a computer-drawn X-ray of the brain itself.

Normally we all experience a certain degree of brain atrophy or shrinkage and brain-weight loss as we get older, due to a decreased number of living brain cells. Alzheimer's disease speeds up the process of cellular shrinkage and cellular death significantly.

CAT scans can measure brain atrophy by indicating space between the skull and the brain related to widespread loss of nerve tissue in the cerebral cortex, or outer covering of the brain. A diagnosis of mild to severe atrophy can be made, depending on the size of the space. Usually, but not always, the greater the degree of dementia, the greater the atrophy.

Inner spaces of the brain, or ventricles, where cerebrospinal fluid normally circulates also increase in size as brain substance decays and is replaced by more fluid. The size of the ventricles may be directly proportional to the degree of dementia.

'Magnetic resonance imaging,' known as *MRI* or *NMR*, is one of the newest head-examining techniques. MRI provides a more detailed picture of the brain than does a CAT scan, and may be ordered if CAT scan results are judged insufficient to make a diagnosis.

Unfortunately, the CAT scan or MRI alone can't provide an absolute diagnosis of Alzheimer's disease. Brain shrinkage is not always apparent. In any case, the only absolute proof is found through brain autopsy following death. But what these tests can do, in conjunction with other tests, is eliminate other possible causes of dementia. Scans can detect brain tumours, cysts, blood clots or haematomas that may have resulted from falls and blows to the head; normal-pressure hydrocephalus, or fluid on the brain; and the stroke activity of multi-infarct dementia.

Pick's disease, a dementia producing lesser degrees of memory loss than Alzheimer's but greater degrees of social and sexually inappropriate behaviour, may also be detected. It is evidenced by severe atrophy in the area of the temporal cortex of the brain. Again, this diagnosis is not conclusive apart from brain autopsy.

In addition to EEG and CAT and MRI scans, *PET* (positron emission tomography) procedures are sometimes done in research facilities. Currently very expensive and rarely used on a routine basis, they may be a future diagnostic tool.

In the PET procedure, radioactive glucose is injected into the brain and studies are done to determine what areas of the brain are able to metabolize the glucose. If someone suffers from Alzheimer's, it is anticipated that there will be certain 'dead' areas in the brain, most notably in the temporal and parietal lobes, where no metabolism will take place.

An even more recent diagnostic tool is called SPECT (single photon emission computerized tomography). SPECT is a procedure researchers hope will help separate treatable types of dementia from irreversible types such as Alzheimer's.

EEGs, CAT and MRI scans, and PET and SPECT

procedures are not painful, but they may be frightening to a person who is confused to begin with. They are usually done in busy hospitals on stretchers or tables that are cold, hard and uncomfortable. If a person fails to relax or is moving around, it may be difficult to get accurate test results. Mild sedation may be ordered prior to the test.

One carer told his wife he was taking her to the beauty parlour. When she arrived at the hospital, she was delighted. The bowl-shaped CAT scanner looked like a giant hair dryer. Once her head was in place, she promptly fell asleep.

Reassurance, going with your loved one to the exam area (something you may have to insist on) and appealing to his or her sense of humour—all may be necessary.

If a person's symptoms are of recent onset, one or more of the foregoing procedures may be done. If symptoms have advanced and progressed for several years, they may not be. But they are all options to consider when you and your relative's doctor are searching for the truth.

CHAPTER THREE
Facing the Facts

Every day at 11:00 a.m. the taxi pulls up in front of the terraced house on Victoria Road. The driver toots, turns off the engine, lights a cigarette and waits for Ralph Murphy, who will soon appear with an umbrella in one hand, shopping bag in the other, and an overcoat thrown over his shoulder. Ralph will suddenly disappear again because he's forgotten to feed the cat, check the rings on the cooker or turn out the lights. But he's seventy-five and entitled to a little memory lapse, thinks the taxi driver.

'Hi ya, Jack.'

'Hi ya, Mr Murphy. The usual, right?'

'Right, Jack. Same time. Same station. Every day. You know me. Can't keep a good man down.'

The taxi inches its way along and finally stops in front of a two-storey brick building surrounded by azaleas. The sign on the door reads, *Riverview Manor Convalescent Home.*

'See you at 2:30,' says Ralph Murphy, handing Jack a five pound note.

'I'll be here,' says the driver. 'Say hello to Mrs Murphy for me.'

'Will do, Jack. Will do.'

Inside, he calls out, 'Harriet, love, I'm here. It's your Ralph.'

Harriet Murphy doesn't turn to acknowledge her husband. Instead, she's looking out her window, pointing with her finger in the general direction of the car park across the street.

'What are you looking at, Honey?'

Harriet doesn't respond. She just continues to point.

'It's about time for dinner. Are you ready, Honey?' asks Ralph.

'Hungry,' says Harriet, looking at her husband for the first time.

'That's my girl.'

Ralph lays his coat and umbrella on the bed, puts his shopping bag in Harriet's lap, grips the handles of her wheelchair, and propels it out the door. They head for the dining room of the nursing home where one tray waits for Harriet and another waits for him, courtesy of the management. Ralph feeds Harriet her dinner and then eats his own, as he has every day for the past four years.

After dinner they'll go out on the patio and look at the birds around the bird table and Ralph will talk to Harriet. He'll tell her stories about the children and grandchilren and great-grandchildren, and they'll look at all the pictures he keeps in the shopping bag.

Then Ralph will wheel Harriet back to her room. He'll kiss her good-bye, tell her he loves her, go out to the desk, joke with the nurses for a few minutes, head for the entrance, get in his waiting taxi and leave.

'How'd it go today, Mr Murphy?' asks Jack.

'Not so good, not so good.'

Jack doesn't say anything more. He knows that today Ralph Murphy just wants to sit back and remember.

It's been a long time since that day in June. Over fifteen years. But Ralph can still remember it as if it were yesterday. You don't forget a thing like that. It's not every day your wife accuses you of being a rapist.

They'd stopped at a motorway service station on their way up to Scotland.

Ralph had gone out to get them a couple of sandwiches and coffee. When he came back to the car, there they were. Harriet, two policemen and a crowd of onlookers.

Before he could open his car door, the questions started.

'Are you the man who claims to be Ralph Murphy?'

'I *am* Ralph Murphy,' he said. 'What's the matter?'

'This woman claims you kidnapped her, raped her and are holding her against her will.'

At that point Ralph started laughing.

'What's so funny?'

'She's my wife,' Ralph repeated. 'My wife. She gets very confused sometimes. Haven't you talked to her?'

'Yes, we did,' said the policeman. 'And you're right. She did seem confused. She told us it was 1931 and a few other things that didn't make much sense. I guess maybe you're right. You act like you're her husband, but you're still going to have to prove it. Is there someone we can call?'

'My son. In Scotland. That's where we were heading.'

So Ralph gave the police the number and they placed the call. His son verified that Ralph was indeed his father, that Harriet was his mother and that, yes, she had been having some memory problems.

'If you've got any more stops to make, Mr Murphy,' said the policeman, 'you might want to cancel your trip. Either that or don't let your wife out of your sight. We believed you. The next time you might not be so lucky.'

The next morning, Ralph and Harriet Murphy headed back to Dorset.

The following week, Ralph made an appointment at the health centre. When he came out of the doctor's surgery two weeks later with a tentative diagnosis of Alzheimer's disease, he knew there'd be no more trips to Scotland. He couldn't deny the decline any longer.

The next few years were hell on earth for him. Harriet's suspicions grew worse. She continued accusing him of molesting her. 'I don't know you. Get out!' she'd scream at him if he tried to come into their bedroom.

He tried to tell Harriet she had an illness when she asked, as she often did, what was wrong with her. 'You have an illness of your mind,' he's say. Then she'd get upset and accuse *him* of being crazy.

Then there was the night she ran away. Luckily he was a light sleeper. He got up and stumbled downstairs when he realized she was gone. He headed for the bridge.

And sure enough, there was Harriet getting ready to jump off the bridge.

This time Ralph was grateful to see the police who were patrolling the area. They helped him get her into the car and take her home.

'You know, you're going to need some help with her,' one of the policemen said.

'I know,' he said.

Three weeks later, Harriet was admitted to Riverview Manor. She hated the place at first. She accused the nurses, the cleaners, even the nursing-home administrator of molesting her, of holding her against her will. And Ralph knew she talked to them about him. What a terrible person he'd been to her. How unfeeling he was for 'dumping her off' like this.

But Harriet was safe. She was clean, dry and fed. She was well taken care of. For that, he was grateful.

'Same time tomorrow, Mr Murphy?' asked the driver, pulling up in front of the terraced house.

'Same time, same station. Thanks, Jack.'

Ralph Murphy got out of the taxi, paid the driver, waved and started up the steps. When he reached the top step he paused, turned around and doubled back to the waiting taxi. He'd forgotten his overcoat.

Blowing Away the Myths

'In short, I believe that the major diseases of human beings have become approachable biological puzzles, ultimately solvable... Strokes and senile dementia, and cancer, and arthritis are not natural aspects of the human condition,' wrote Dr. Lewis Thomas in *The Medusa and the Snail*. In addition to chronic and dementing diseases, another impediment we need to rid ourselves of is myths.

In relation to dementia in general and Alzheimer's in particular, many myths abound. There's a lot of fiction mixed in with the facts, largely arising out of fear and/or lack of knowledge.

Myth Number 1: All old people get senile.
All confused people age, but all people who age do not become confused. Chronology is not synonymous with confusion.

In actual fact, only about five per cent of all people over the age of sixty-five are severely impaired intellectually due to dementia. An additional ten per cent may be mildly to moderately impaired.

That leaves eighty-five percent of people over sixty-five with minds that, intellectually speaking, function very well indeed.

Any sign of forgetfulness in our loved ones or even ourselves should not trigger a panic attack. Just because you forgot where you put your car keys, missed an appointment with your dentist, or can't remember where you stored last summer's picnic supplies does not mean you're in the early stages of Alzheimer's. Isolated instances of forgetfulness may simply be related to information overload or the natural memory loss we all experience from time to time.

As we grow up we grow old, and this ageing process includes our brains. Any one of us, if we live into our seventies, eighties or nineties, will undoubtedly experience a small degree of forgetfulness. That's because the senile plaques and neurofibrillary tangles that are so characteristic of Alzheimer's are also present in normal ageing brains. But, unlike the plaques and tangles of Alzheimer's, they are scattered throughout the brain and are fewer in number. Although they can contribute to occasional memory lapses, especially when we're under stress, they don't result in full-blown dementia for most of us.

Myth Number 2: If you keep your mind active and read more books, you won't get Alzheimer's.

Neither Alzheimer's disease nor any of the other incurable dementias can be prevented or staved off by keeping your mind and body active in your youth. Alzheimer's is no respecter of persons. It knows no social, sexual, ethnic or educational boundaries.

Myth Number 3: Alzheimer's disease is contagious.

Alzheimer's is *not* contagious. You can't catch it like you can AIDS or the flu. It's not bloodborne or airborne; it is related to a specific disease process.

Myth Number 4: There are many treatments for Alzheimer's disease.

To date, there are no recommended treatments for Alzheimer's disease. There *are*, however, many false prophets in the world eager to take our hard-earned money. They advocate any number of cures and correctives and sometimes even try to pinpoint a cause. Their bogus remedies range from massive doses of megavitamins to various herbal remedies. The claims of alternative medicine must be examined cautiously.

Myth Number 5: The confusion could easily be cleared up if the blood flowed better. I've heard there are pills you can take that dilate the blood vessels.

Some drugs, called *vasodilators*, increase the diameter of the blood vessels in the brain. Alzheimer's, however, is not a vascular disease, and many doctors believe that vasodilators can in fact be harmful to elderly people with Alzheimer's type dementia. Vasodilators also dilate peripheral blood vessels in the arms and legs and can actually reduce the pressure available for adequate cerebral blood flow. Decreased blood pressure, such as that which frequently occurs when a person suddenly stands up, can result in lightheadedness and falls, especially in Alzheimer's victims who have difficulty maintaining balance and co-ordination. If used at all, vasodilators should be used with caution and carefully evaluated by both doctor and carer.

The Aluminium Question

Although it has been known for some time that higher-than-normal concentrations of aluminium salts have been found in the brain cells of people who suffered from Alzheimer's and other dementias, most researchers believed that excess aluminium was the result, not the cause of the disease. However, there is a growing amount of circumstantial evidence linking aluminium with Alzheimer's disease.

The following findings are among reasons for concern:

- Aluminium is one of the few substances known to cause brain tangles and memory loss when injected into certain animals. The tangles are similar, though not identical, to those which occur in man.

- Aluminium was identified as the cause of 'dialysis dementia' suffered by some patients undergoing dialysis for kidney disease. This condition was prevented by removing aluminium from the dialysis fluid.

- A recent survey suggested that rates of Alzheimer's Disease were approximately one and a half times more frequent in districts with higher levels of aluminium in the water, compared with those in which it was low or absent.

Aluminium is one of the most common metals in our environment. We are daily exposed to its chemical forms in the food we eat, the water, tea and coffee we drink, the medications we take, and even the deodorants we use. Some people also experience occupational exposure to dust containing aluminium or aluminium compounds.

None of this is proof that aluminium contributes to the degenerative changes which cause Alzheimer's Disease. However, it may be that some people are more at risk because of genetic or other factors and would benefit from a reduction in their intake of aluminium. For the present, you may feel that it is prudent to avoid foods containing aluminium additives and to use non-aluminium pans and utensils, particularly for cooking acidic foods which are known to leach more aluminium from the pan.

Further research is needed before any definite conclusions can be drawn. It is helpful to remember that even if a clear link is found with Alzheimer's, the risk from any past or present exposure to aluminium is still small.

When we see our loved one deteriorating before our eyes, it's only natural to want to grasp at any available straw if there's even a remote possibility it might help alleviate some of the symptoms of Alzheimer's and slow the disease process.

But it's also natural and in our best interests to ask questions before investing our money for something that, in the long run, could make the condition worse.

When in doubt about an advertised home-remedy or an expensive treatment offered in some out-of-the-way place, the best thing to do is nothing—until you have called or written to the Alzheimer's Disease Society (see Appendix D) and requested information. They can also give you information about legitimate experimental drug trials being conducted with Alzheimer's sufferers. There are a number in progress.

There is, at present, no treatment or cure for Alzheimer's disease. But there is hope. Alzheimer's is not a normal process of ageing. It is a disease, a deviation from the norm. And, as we've learned through experience over the years, all diseases *are* solvable biological puzzles that may one day reveal to us the reasons for their existence.

For the sake of our loved ones and for future generations, we need to pray that day will come soon.

Don't Deny the Decline

> My aunt became very frustrated. She knew there was something desperately wrong with her, and she would sit in her chair and whimper a lot. She always had this sad, sad look. And she thought—and we thought—she was losing her mind.

> There were other things, as I look back, that I should have noticed about my wife. In November of 1976 she wanted to have our wills made out. She kept insisting. I wonder if she knew something then that I didn't know or even suspect?

> 'What's the use?' I remember my husband saying to me

when he first started to lose his memory. 'What's the
point of living?'

People in the early stages of Alzheimer's disease need all
the support they can get from family, friends, relatives and
the community. They need to be assured they aren't going
crazy, that life is not over for them, that they are still loved
and accepted.

Denial is a very common reaction to the diagnosis of
Alzheimer's and to the initial symptoms of memory loss,
even before a diagnosis is made.

We may deny because our loved one's behaviour doesn't
fit our expectations of a disease. Most people are used to
equating illness with observable signs. People with Alzheimer's usually look healthy and alert. They may, in fact, have
considerably more energy than we do. Instead of blaming a
disease, we attribute their confusion to the myth of senility,
or to various changes that occur in mid-to-late life:

> I didn't realize there was anything wrong with my
> husband for a very long time. He was always so healthy
> and still is, even though he's been diagnosed with
> Alzheimer's for over four years.
>   In the beginning I just thought his memory pro-
> blems were part of his ageing, and I guess I thought
> that if your mind was slipping badly your body should
> be falling apart too. His wasn't.

> My mother was always a little eccentric and a bit of a
> loner. She just seemed to get more eccentric as the
> years progressed. She withdrew from life more and
> more after she retired. But she looked so healthy we
> didn't worry about it

Actually we thought Mum was going through
menopause. She seemed to have all the signs and
symptoms, though they were a bit exaggerated.

We may also deny out of shame or embarrassment. In
past generations, families with relatives who were mentally
ill or mentally handicapped kept them 'in the cupboard', so
to speak. They never talked about them outside the immediate family. And, in some cases, people literally kept
their relatives in the cupboard.

For some families, there's still a stigma attached to
mental illness and mental retardation. This stigma can
carry over into the way we feel about a loved one with
dementia.

We may also think people outside our immediate family
won't understand our relative's bizarre behaviour and will
judge us. We're sure they're saying, 'There's Harry again,
acting strange. Why doesn't Virginia *do* something?'

So, embarrassed by an Alzheimer's sufferer's behaviour,
we try to protect everyone involved from potentially embarrassing situations:

In the beginning we didn't know what was happening
to Dad. When he started acting strange in front of
other people, we were embarrassed. We tried to cover
it up because of our embarrassment. Actually we ourselves were immature.

My wife would make a fool of herself in restaurants.
She would say suggestive things to the waiters and
waitresses. One time she even pinched a waiter on the
bottom. I was embarrassed to death and apologized for
her behaviour. Then, finally, I stopped taking her
places altogether.

We may deny because the truth is too painful to accept:

My daughter will sit next to her mother for hours at a time now and her mother won't speak to her, won't recognize her. I know it's hard on her. Awfully hard.

My daughter didn't want to accept her mother's illness in the first place. The doctor told her, 'You've got to start accepting it. You've got to tell your children what's going on. It's not going to get better.'

And the doctor was right. It didn't.

There's also a natural tendency for us to want to preserve the lives and livelihoods of our loved ones for as long as possible:

I wrote my husband's cover letters for him when he was applying for jobs. I knew it was stupid. He wouldn't have been able to do any of those jobs anyway. But I didn't want to see him give up. It was denial I guess. Either that or blind faith.

There was a lot of denial on my part. I didn't want things to end. I didn't want him not to be able to drive any more. His self-esteem was so shaken anyway that I just wanted him to do what he could for as long as possible... So I let him drive, even when I knew he wasn't safe on the road. And I prayed a lot.

It's very easy for us as carers to deny because our loved ones deny as well. They can make tremendous efforts to compensate for their failing faculties:

I'm sure my husband had Alzheimer's for several

years before he was diagnosed. But he was always so good at concealing his memory loss. He joked about it a lot, about how when he got older he just had so many more things to think about that it was easy to have more things to forget. I thought that that made sense.

Sometimes health professionals don't help our situation and, at times, can even make it worse. Doctors aren't immune to the myth of senility:

For three years my husband told the doctors he was having trouble with his memory. For three years the doctors kept telling him, 'Everybody does when they get to a certain age.'
Finally things got so bad my husband couldn't perform his job. They finally started to listen.

In the case of Alzheimer's, we might sometimes feel as if we'd rather not know. But ignorance is not really bliss. To be forewarned is to be forearmed. There are six good reasons why, sooner or later, we have to stop denying.

Six Reasons to Face the Facts

Information drives away fear. Early recognition of Alzheimer's disease can help us deal with our own fears more realistically. One reason Alzheimer's is so fearful is that it makes us feel out of control. We cannot prevent it, arrest it or stop it. One of the best ways to allay this fear is through knowledge and understanding of the disease itself. There are many reputable sources from which we can get reliable information. The more information we have to draw from, the better able we'll be to cope with this devastating disease.

One of the best sources of reliable information is the

Alzheimer's Disease Society. The Society was founded in 1979 and many regional branches have been formed as well as relatives' support groups in most parts of Britain. There are Alzheimer's associations in over twenty countries.

The Alzheimer's Disease Society has several purposes:

- It supports research into the causes and possible cures for Alzheimer's disease and other forms of dementia.

- It helps organize carer support groups to assist, encourage and educate carers.

- It sponsors educational programmes and provides written and audio-visual information on Alzheimer's disease and related disorders for both professional and nonprofessional carers.

- It advocates for carers and people with Alzheimer's disease in areas of legislation— both locally and nationally.

The earlier we are aware of information and available resources, the less likely we are to be faced with a full-blown crisis later, when management problems become increasingly difficult and we need outside help.

Our loved ones must be kept safe. Denial can become dangerous—especially for the loved one living alone, as many people do in the early stages of Alzheimer's.

If our loved one is in danger of falling, of setting the house on fire because of forgetfulness, or of wandering off and getting lost, the time has come to actively intervene, whether we want to or not. Independence is not something that can be preserved indefinitely for someone with Alzheimer's.

This recognition of danger may not mean suddenly uprooting loved ones and moving them in with us, but it will mean providing for their safety in practical ways, such as hiring home-care workers or a live-in companion.

Our loved ones may benefit from ongoing research. To date, there are no marketable drugs that claim to treat Alzheimer's, but many carers credit experimental drug trials with alleviating some of the symptoms of the disease. Drug trials are being conducted all over the world at various hospitals and research centres. The earlier the diagnosis, the greater the chance an Alzheimer's sufferer will qualify for a programme should he or she wish to do so. Local or regional support groups or chapters can help identify various locations where studies are going on. The Alzheimer's Disease Society can also provide information.

The entire family should play a role in caring. Alzheimer's disease is a family affair. In most instances spouses, siblings, children, grandchildren, great-grandchildren and an assortment of in-laws are involved. All have roles and responsibilities when it comes to caring, and open communication early in the course of the disease is important to ensure that the burden of caring is shared.

Financial arrangements must be made. Alzheimer's not only bankrupts the mind; it can also take its toll on family finances and savings accounts. There are many hidden costs involved in caring at home and the carer's potential for earning is obviously affected. Residential care, home care and respite care can all be expensive so it is best to explore all options. It is important to be aware of the benefits available to carers and to claim those to which you are entitled.

Legal advice may need to be sought, whether through the Citizens Advice Bureau, Law Centre, a private solicitor or the Court of Protection. At the earliest possible stage, carers need to consider obtaining an Enduring Power of Attorney enabling them to take charge of their loved one's affairs when it becomes necessary to do so. It is also worth knowing that sufferers from dementia should be exempt from paying Council Tax.

The Alzheimer's Disease Society has published information sheets on Welfare Rights, and Financial and Legal Arrangements, and can also offer advice relevant to specific situations.

The future must be planned. An early diagnosis of Alzheimer's can give both you and your loved one time to think together about what you would do if you had a future with many long years ahead of you. Then, think about living out the future *now*. For example, you may want to take early retirement or go on that trip you've been putting off.

Memory loss in the early stages of Alzheimer's does not mean people are incapable of making any rational decisions. On the contrary, they need to be involved in planning their own future to as great a degree as possible. This may even include the difficult decision of whether or not they want to be resuscitated should they have a cardiac or respiratory arrest in the final stages of their illness.

Alzheimer's is a fatal disease. It's been called a terminal illness that results in a slow death of the mind.

As with any terminal illness, it is a natural initial reaction to deny. Our denial of Alzheimer's disease acts as a cushion. It softens the blow to protect us early on from the emotional pain and distress we might otherwise not be able to handle. Yet finally to admit that our loved ones are experiencing more than 'just a little memory loss' can be a relief. For them and for us.

One carer I interviewed told me about an experience of her young son. They were at a family picnic on a beach near a group of people who suffered from mild to severe mental and physical disabilities.

'A lot of the other children seemed afraid of them,' said the carer. 'Their behaviour was a bit different, and many of the children seemed to be intentionally avoiding them. They'd back away. But not my son. He said, "Look, Mummy. There are some sick people from the hospital."'

'My son certainly wasn't afraid of them. He walked right up to their group, reached out, shook some of their hands and introduced himself. I think it had a lot to do with him spending so much time with his grandmother who has Alzheimer's. He's used to being around people whose behaviour is different.'

We can learn a lot from this young child. As carers we need to have the courage to walk up to the disease, look it squarely in the eye, and shake it by the hand. We need to say, 'I am not afraid of you, and I'm not going to deny your existence.' And we need to say to our loved one, 'I love you. I'm not ashamed of your behaviour. We'll fight this disease together.' It's this kind of realistic and healthy attitude that can carry us beyond the inevitable denial and move us into acceptance.

If you are a carer, write to the Alzheimer's Disease Society and request an order form of available information. If you don't belong to a support group that gets the Society's regular newsletter, ask to be put on their mailing list. The address of the Alzheimer's Disease Society can be found in Appendix D.

In addition to information that can be ordered through the Alzheimer's Disease Society, there are many other useful resources available. A number of them are listed in Appendix D.

CHAPTER FOUR

What's Happening Upstairs?

Well, here they were again. Four o'clock on a Friday afternoon and headed for the café. Precisely at three, Anna had started pacing up and down, up and down in the kitchen at home, repeating the same old question, 'When are we going? When are we going? When are we going to go?' The same question she'd asked nearly every afternoon for the past six months.

Sam couldn't understand it.

His daughter had tried to explain it to him. 'It's part of her disease, Dad. She can't help it. People with Alzheimer's often repeat themselves, over and over again.'

Damnedest disease he'd ever seen. Why couldn't she have got diabetes or broken her hip? That you could live with. But no, Anna had to go and get senile.

Funny thing about it was she'd always been so clever. Always had her head in a book. Did the taxes. Kept the cheque-book. Paid the bills.

Now Sam had to do all those things. All those things he didn't like. He'd never had a head for figures. Anna was the brains of the outfit.

He sure didn't expect retirement to be like this. They

were supposed to be able to relax and enjoy life after forty years of working in the factory. Both of them. Forty years apiece. They'd retired at the same time, five years ago. They'd planned to move to Canada.

Canada! Ha! Anna couldn't even go around the block without getting lost. Imagine what would happen if they went to Canada! She'd probably wind up in some remote place with Sam searching for her. They'd both die of exposure.

She'd forgotten how to cook, too. Anna had always been such a good cook. Nothing fancy—just your basic meat and potatoes. But good meat and good potatoes. And always ready when Sam was hungry. They used to love to eat. After work, Anna would cook a big meal, then maybe they'd watch the news on TV, then go over to their daughter's house and spend some time with the grandchildren. They did that, that is, until their daughter's husband got transferred to Germany. That ended that.

Now Sam and Anna didn't eat at home much any more except when Sam did the cooking, and Sam hated to cook. Never could work out how to poach an egg just right or even make a good cup of coffee. And he did like his poached eggs and coffee.

Cooking, cleaning, paying the bills. All these things Sam had to do now, if he wanted them done at all. 'Too much,' he thought. 'Too much.'

'When we gonna get there? When we gonna get there?'

Anna snapped Sam out of his musings as the car pulled up at the café, seven miles from home.

'We're here, love, we're here.'

'Good. Let's eat,' said Anna.

Sam opened his door, went around the car, and helped Anna out. She brushed off his hand as if it were a fly and ran up the steps of the café.

'Hi, Sam. Hi, Anna. Want a menu?' asked Bill, the owner.

'No. You know we don't need one,' Sam said as they sat down in the booths by the row of windows.

'Menu. Menu. Menu,' said Anna.

'Oh, all right. Give us a menu. She can look. I'll order.'

'Looks like she's been putting on some weight again. You too. Guess that's good, huh, Sam?' said Bill.

'Yeah,' said Sam. 'Anna never eats much when we're home. Guess she doesn't like my cooking. Guess that's why you're still in business, because of people like us.'

'So what'll it be today?'

'The usual. Two egg and chips. Two coffees.'

'No,' said Anna, peering over her menu and glaring at her husband. 'No. No. No.'

'Oh, I almost forgot,' said Sam. 'And two big pieces of apple pie.'

Anna smiled.

'Give me the menu, Anna,' said Sam.

'No. No. No. No.'

'That's all right, Sam. She can keep it.'

'Thanks, Bill. Give her something to look at while we're waiting. Give her something to read. She always did so like to read. I wonder what went wrong? What went wrong?'

'My mind is all mixed up. Like this,' my mother once said to me, holding up a tangled purple strand of wool she was attempting to crochet into one of her famous afghans.

Mixed up. Tangled. Like a skein of wool that's slowly being unravelled by a precocious kitten. That's a fairly accurate picture of what happens to someone suffering from Alzheimer's disease.

Alzheimer's is not a normal result of ageing. It's related to a specific disease process. Very distinct pathological changes take place in the brain. Under a microscope these changes *do* resemble a tangled skein of wool.

When someone we love is 'all mixed up' because of a

confusion-causing disease like Alzheimer's, it's important to have as much information as possible to better understand the disease process.

But to understand what goes wrong, we first need to take a look at what's normal. How are our brains supposed to work? How are they structured? Just what *does* go on in our heads, anyway?

The brain is, quite literally, the headquarters for the rest of the body. It's the main office, the control tower, the central meeting place for a vast network of nerves that control all our conscious activity and affect our unconscious actions as well.

The brain isn't much to look at. On the surface it rather resembles a three-pound walnut. But beneath the grey and convoluted exterior of the brain is housed a complex information storage and retrieval system that is responsible for memory, thoughts, language, behaviour and emotions.

The brain consists of three main parts: the cerebrum, or large brain; the cerebellum, or small brain; and the brain stem.

The *cerebrum* fills nearly the entire brain cavity and consists of two cerebral hemispheres covered by a grey outer covering called the *cerebral cortex*. This 'grey matter' is associated with our higher mental functions.

The *cerebellum*, located at the back of the brain cavity and below the cerebrum, is responsible for balance and co-ordinates muscular activity.

The *brain stem* connects the brain to the spinal column and controls the vital functions of breathing and circulation.

To illustrate how a normal brain works, and to better understand what goes wrong when a person becomes afflicted with Alzheimer's, let's look at one specific activity our brains are engaged in every day: making decisions.

The brain, like the rest of our organs, is made up of billions of microscopic cells. In the brain these cells are called *neurons*. Each neuron has a round cell body inside it called a *cell nucleus*.

Each cell nucleus sends out short, branching shoots called *dendrites* through one side of its neuron. These free-floating branches are called *dendrite receivers*. The other side of the neuron branches out into *transmitter dendrites* that are gathered together and funneled through a long, threadlike structure called an *axon*.

Let's say we decide to visit a neighbour.

We can't do this with our feet alone. They won't move by themselves. We have to communicate our desire to take a walk to our brain. Our brain passes the message on to our feet.

The message to walk to the neighbour's house is transmitted by an electrical impulse originating in one or more of the cell nuclei. This impulse passes through the transmitter dendrites, through the axon, and on into the terminal shoots or branches that pop out through the end of the axon.

At the end of each cluster of terminal transmitter-dendrite branches is a space or gap called a *synapse*.

Once the electrical impulse from our message reaches this synapse, it somehow has to bridge it and communicate with the dendrite receivers of a neighbouring neuron. The impulse does this by stimulating the release of chemicals called *neurotransmitters*. There are many different neurotransmitters. (One important one is acetylcholine. Acetylcholine is believed to be responsible for or plays a major role in thinking and remembering, and is especially important in the processing of recent or short-term memory.)

Once the neurotransmitters are released, they pass through the synaptic space and are attached to the surface of the dendrite receivers at specific locations known as *receptors*. This stimulates the release of a high-energy chemical that switches on the electrical impulse in the next neuron along the path.

The brain then tells our feet to take a walk.

This process of message transmission in the brain is indeed beautiful, rather like a well-crocheted afghan. It is evidence that the brain, like the rest of us, is wonderfully made, a complex creation knit together by a loving and imaginative creator, enabling us to function in amazing ways.

What Goes Wrong?

I tried to explain it to him so he would understand. I told my husband that having Alzheimer's was like having a car with its wires disconnected. I told him they hadn't figured out a way yet to reconnect the wires in his brain. He seemed to accept that.

_____

I think my son described it best. He said there's a whole lot of switches in the brain and, one by one, they go.

_____

My husband started acting really strangely the summer of 1979. By November he was worse. I tried to get him to go to the doctor but he refused.

He would always shower in the morning. If he was active, he'd also shower at night. But that fall he let himself go and didn't shower at all. He wouldn't even change his clothes. He seemed deeply depressed.

If I said anything to him about what he was doing, or not doing, he would get angry. I knew there was something wrong, and he knew there was something wrong, but he wouldn't admit it.

One day our son happened to be visiting. He said, 'You know, some of the things you're doing aren't *you*.

Don't you think Mother ought to make an appointment for you to see a doctor?'

I guess my husband needed to hear it from our son, because he came back into the house later that day and said, 'You're right. I've got to see a doctor. I've got to find out what's wrong with me.'

The year was 1906. The country was Germany.

He was a psychiatrist and neuropathologist. She was a middle-aged housewife experiencing profound memory loss, disorientation, confusion, depression, insomnia and hallucinations.

She, his patient, died in a nursing home at age fifty-five. He decided to conduct an autopsy.

When Dr. Alois Alzheimer looked in his microscope and, using a special silver stain, examined a slice of his patient's brain tissue, he discovered two startling abnormalities, inside and outside the brain cells.

Tissue lying inside the cell bodies or nuclei of neurons exhibited an abnormally high number of fine nerve fibres, or filaments, twisted around each other. Dr. Alzheimer called these twisted fibres *neurofibrillary tangles*.

He also saw unusually high numbers of fibrous plaques located between brain cells, composed of degenerating terminal dendrites or burned-out nerve endings that surrounded fibrous waste products of amyloid protein. These abnormalities were known as *senile* or *neuritic plaques*. They had been identified before in the autopsied brain tissue of much older people.

For many years after 1906, it was believed that this characteristic tangle and plaque configuration occurred primarily in people under the age of sixty-five; Alzheimer's disease was thought to be a 'pre-senile dementia.'

Anyone exhibiting signs of confusion after age sixty-five was simply labeled 'senile' or was said to have a chronic organic brain syndrome, more commonly known as COBS.

This senility of old age was universally blamed on faulty blood circulation or so-called hardening of the arteries, and it was thought to be due to an atherosclerotic process of cholesterol build-up in the arteries of the brain.

But in succeeding years, research finally caught up with reality. In the 1960s, as British researchers began comparing the brains of younger, deceased dementia victims with those of older victims, the electron microscope proved what many had suspected all along: the primary cause of dementia-like symptoms in both younger and older victims was, in fact, one and the same. And it wasn't as rare a phenomenon as previously thought.

Investigators believed the fibrous plaques and neurofibrillary tangles disrupted the passage of neurochemical signals between neurons, resulting in memory loss and impaired thought processes.

In general, the greater the number of plaques, tangles and associated cellular death, the greater the degree of disturbance in intellectual function. These changes in the brain took place over time and were responsible for the progressive nature of the disease. And while there was a decrease in blood flow to the brain in victims of Alzheimer's disease, this decrease was not caused by atherosclerosis but by brain-cell death brought on by the Alzheimer's process.

In the 1970s researchers discovered another abnormality associated with Alzheimer's disease, one specifically related to neurochemical changes and the neurotransmitter acetylcholine, normally manufactured in the brain by an enzyme known as *choline acetyltransferase.*

In autopsied brain tissue of people who have the characteristic plaques and tangles, choline acetyltransferase and acetylcholine are missing or present in decreased amounts.

Without the stimulus for neurotransmission, signals (messages) are unable to move across the synaptic gap from neuron to neuron. When nerve cells can't communicate with each other, trouble occurs.

This neurochemical loss, as well as the appearance of plaques and tangles, occurs primarily in two areas of the brain: the cortex and the hippocampus.

The cortex, or outer surface of the brain's cerebrum, is composed of those cell bodies that enable us to reason, remember and speak. In addition to experiencing the neurochemical loss, the cortex of Alzheimer's victims usually shrinks or atrophies, decreasing the brain's surface area.

The hippocampus is a small cluster of cells located in the temporal lobe. It is extremely important to short-term memory function and is also part of the limbic system. This system, activated by motivated behaviour and arousal, influences both the hormones and the autonomic motor system, which controls involuntary body functions. It has been called 'the seat of our emotions.'

What is actually responsible for the development of plaques, tangles and the death of acetylcholine-producing cells is unknown. Researchers around the world are exploring possible causes or combinations of causes that include genetic factors, a slow virus, abnormalities in the immune system, infectious agents, toxic substances in the environment, metabolic deficits, and abnormalities in DNA repair. Appendix C includes a more detailed overview of research related to causation.

Today Alzheimer's and the senility associated with old age are categorized as one and the same process. They are generally referred to as pre-senile dementia or senile dementia of the Alzheimer's type, depending on the age of onset. The former usually occurs before age sixty-five; the latter, after.

Our brains are indeed awesomely and wonderfully made, but sometimes things do go wrong with this complex computer that controls us, things we struggle to understand.

Seeing the Symptoms

'Hindsight is always better than foresight,' acknowledged one carer. 'I think the reason I didn't see my wife's symptoms earlier was because I was with her all the time. The changes were so subtle, so gradual.'

Probably the most remarkable thing about the very early stages of Alzheimer's disease is its unremarkableness. Signs and symptoms seem to creep up and take us unaware, surprising both us and our loved ones. With the passage of time, the mental and physical deterioration of Alzheimer's becomes more and more pronounced.

While no two people progress at the same rate or according to the same exact pattern, there are some characteristic behaviour and personality changes peculiar to each stage of the illness. Knowing what these changes are can help you promote a better quality of life for both yourself and your loved one. Understanding the signs and symptoms of Alzheimer's is a crucial key to caring.

Two to four years is the average length of the first stage of Alzheimer's. The initial symptoms of Alzheimer's may include any or all of the following:

Memory loss. Recent events are forgotten. The ability to concentrate, learn new things and process new information is progressively lost. Bills go unpaid or are paid several times. Checking accounts are overdrawn when the person has trouble adding, subtracting and balancing a chequebook. The names of known and loved persons may also be forgotten.

People with Alzheimer's often compensate, initially, by writing notes to themselves. But as the disease progresses, they no longer remember the notes. People frequently deny experiencing these symptoms as they struggle to preserve their self-esteem and identity.

Confusion and disorientation. Confusion is often related to place and time. People with Alzheimer's sometimes get lost on their way somewhere, or they will arrive at a place and not know where they are or how to get home. The day and month are forgotten as well.

Speech and language disturbances. There may be a progressive inability to name objects or to end sentences. The person searches for words and phrases. Wrong words and phrases are substituted for the forgotten right ones, a condition known as *confabulation.* *Circumlocution* may also occur, where more words than necessary are used to express an idea.

Impaired judgement. There's a lack of insight and a growing inability to discriminate, understand and follow directions. Driving is progressively impaired; the person may fail to stop at junctions or go the wrong way on one-way streets. The ability to read is retained but not the ability to understand what is read.

Difficulty completing familiar tasks. It becomes increasingly difficult to cook, clean, engage in familiar hobbies, hold down a job. Routine activities of daily living go through a process of 'unlearning.' For example, the ability to tie shoes, button a blouse or shirt, or make a cup of coffee may be impaired.

Personality and mood changes. Depression frequently accompanies the early stage of Alzheimer's. There may be listlessness, apathy, suspiciousness, paranoia, social withdrawal and episodes of crying. Conversely, there may be restlessness, anxiety, agitation and feelings of 'going crazy'. On the one hand people deny the severity of their symptoms, while on the other, they recognize that something's wrong.

Carelessness and neglect. Personal hygiene can become a problem, and people may appear careless or unkempt. They may neglect to bathe, brush their teeth, change or wash their clothes. They simply may have forgotten how.

Following a diagnosis, carers usually ask their GP, 'How long do we have? How many months or years?' There is always a need to know.

The time from the onset of Alzheimer's to the person's death varies greatly. It may be a few years or over twenty, depending on any number of other health-related factors. Generally speaking, the younger a person is, the faster the progression and deterioration.

Facing the Second Stage

'There are some lucid moments, but they are few and far between and they seem to be getting farther and farther away from each other,' reported one carer whose wife had been diagnosed with Alzheimer's five years earlier.

This can be called stage two. As the disease progresses, stage one symptoms intensify. Memory loss becomes more profound. Behaviour becomes more disturbing, bizarre and unpredictable. This second stage of Alzheimer's may last for two to ten years.

We need to keep in mind that not all victims of Alzheimer's will experience the same symptoms, but there are some behaviour changes common to dementia.

Continued and progressive memory loss. Past events as well as recent ones may no longer be remembered. The ability to engage in familiar hobbies or carry out even the routine activities of daily living, such as bathing, dressing and toileting, is impaired.

Progressive to complete disorientation and confusion. Our loved ones may lose their ability to recognize people, including family members. They may not recognize their own reflection in a mirror. They may forget the names and uses of familiar objects. They may wander off and get lost, or they may even get lost in their own homes.

Speech, communication and language disorders. People with second-stage Alzheimer's are progressively unable to express themselves and to complete sentences. The repetition of words, questions and phrases is common. Speech may become garbled or very slow.

Catastrophic reactions. These may include pronounced mood swings or personality changes including outbursts of anger, increased suspiciousness or paranoia and even episodes of physical violence, usually short-lived.

Wandering, restlessness and pacing. Restless wandering often occurs at night or in the late afternoon, around dusk. Repetitious movements, such as finger or foot tapping, lip smacking and constant chewing motions, may increase.

Various behaviour problems. There may be hallucinations or delusions of being persecuted. People with Alzheimer's frequently hide and hoard things and may tear the house apart looking for 'lost' items. There may be inappropriate sexual and social behaviour with marked social withdrawal.

Physical signs. Motor activity may be affected; many people in the second stage progressively lose their ability to engage in activities requiring hand and finger co-ordination. Opening a tin with a tin-opener, buttoning a shirt, tying a shoelace, hammering a nail—all could be affected.

Occasionally there is muscle twitching or jerking. People may tend to lose their balance and fall as co-ordination becomes impaired. Eating and elimination problems manifest themselves.

The following chapters highlight some of the more common and difficult management problems carers have identified, along with suggestions on how to deal with these problems in the varying stages of the disease.

PART TWO

CARING FOR YOUR LOVED ONE

*We can do no great things—only small
things with great love.*

MOTHER TERESA

CHAPTER FIVE

When Memory Starts to Fade

'The gifts of God for the people of God. Take them in remembrance that Christ died for you, and feed on him in your hearts by faith, with thanksgiving.'

Father Joe walked slowly down the row of communicants, pausing before each of his parishioners to say the familiar words. 'The body of Christ, the bread of heaven. The body of Christ, the bread of heaven. The body of Christ, the bread of heaven.'

When he came to the last kneeling person, he paused and smiled. Here was Mary again. Just as she had been for the past eight months.

Mary. A seventy-five-year-old woman who never married, and a founder member of the church. A Sunday school teacher for forty years until she was sixty-five, at which time she told everyone she was tired, retired, and ready to relax. 'You folks take over,' said Mary. 'I'll sit and enjoy church.'

Mary, whose habits the past eight months had become rather unusual. She had developed a weekly pattern of bringing her luggage—two overstuffed suitcases held together with string and adhesive tape—to church. She'd even carry them up to the altar and set them down, one on each side of her. Father Joe once asked Mary where she was going with her suitcases. Mary glared at him and told him it was none of his business.

Today, Mary wasn't exactly dressed for church, not for church on a warm summer morning, at any rate. She had on her bulky grey overcoat with the unraveling hem and what appeared to be several layers of thick wool stockings. A pair of fur-lined boots graced her feet. One toe stuck out through a hole.

It wasn't as if Mary had to wear these clothes, thought Father Joe. The ladies of the church had offered to take her shopping. They'd even purchased some new summer clothes for her and had delivered them in person. But Mary wouldn't let them in the house, telling them she didn't accept charity and to please give the clothes to the poor. 'I'm fine,' Mary insisted. 'Fine.'

And Mary *was* fine, to a point. The Meals-on-Wheels programme delivered a hot lunch to her—so she was at least eating a balanced diet. But Mary never let the volunteers in the house, insisting they leave the food on the front step. By every morning the previous day's meals had disappeared, and the dirty dishes were back on the step.

The district nurses were aware of Mary's situation and were also trying to help. They sent a home help to clean her house, but Mary wouldn't let her inside. She insisted, through the keyhole, that she was fine. 'My house is clean,' she told the woman.

'It sure didn't smell fine and clean through the keyhole!' the home help told her supervisor. 'But what could I do?'

Today, though, Mary's clothes and Mary's house really didn't matter. Mary was here in church, and she was ready to receive communion.

As Father Joe bent down to place the wafer in Mary's mouth, he could detect the odour of urine floating up and mingling its ammonia with the aroma of burning incense.

But Mary wasn't aware of this. Her eyes were closed in an attitude of prayer. Her mouth was open to receive the wafer. And her hands gripped the handles of her two packed suitcases.

Of all of us gathered here today, thought Father Joe, Mary is probably the most prepared to enter the heavenly kingdom.

The Faces of Memory Loss

Several weeks before I completed the final draft of the first edition of this book, the father of a member of our support group died. I went to the viewing at the funeral parlour, where my friend and I stood next to her father's casket, talking about the final, emotionally charged days of his life.

As I was about to leave, my friend turned to me and said, 'Be sure to tell people that Alzheimer's is more than a little memory loss. It's not just forgetting names or how to balance your cheque-book. It's forgetting everything, eventually. Everything you ever did that was important to who you were as a person. Everyone you've ever known. Write about that. People need to know.'

My friend was right. People do need to know. For with knowledge comes understanding and the ability to empathize with carers faced with a responsibility that may last anywhere from one to over twenty years. As carers ourselves, we need knowledge and understanding to be able to deal with the many faces of Alzheimer's, especially the many faces of memory loss.

My own mother was an artist. Not a professional artist, but an artist nonetheless. My most vivid childhood memories are of Mum sitting in her living-room rocking chair each evening after tea, in front of an old easel my father made, surrounded by little tubes of oil paint or boxes of pastels. Mum was always in the middle of a painting project.

Later in life my mother packed up her paints and pastels and switched to crocheting. With her artist's eye she wove thousands of granny squares into dozens of beautiful afghans. When she first started having symptoms of Alzheimer's, she continued to crochet. In fact, her afghans were one of the first signs that anything was wrong.

I came home for a visit one Christmas and Mum had one of her latest creations spread out on the bed. It basically looked normal, much the same as all her other variegated blue-and-white afghans. This one, however, also contained a few isolated squares of green and white. When I mentioned it, my mother just shrugged. 'Looks okay to me,' I remember her saying. That did not show an artist's appraising eye, and it was not her usual attitude. My mother always liked her afghans to be perfect, and she would tear them apart and start them over if they weren't.

As the months passed, Mum continued to crochet, but the granny squares gradually became circles, then chains and, finally, bunches of tangled wool. Unlike many people with Alzheimer's who become frustrated with the loss of their ability to continue to engage in well-loved hobbies, Mum seemed content to do what she could and was generally oblivious to the fact that her abilities were deteriorating.

My husband forgot how to dress himself. He couldn't figure out how to button his shirt, tie his shoes or buckle his belt. He just couldn't seem to figure out what went where.

Dad had a colostomy and had always done his own irrigating, but it got to the point where he couldn't remember how to do it. So my mother started to do it for him. Then, eventually, the district nurse came in because Dad wouldn't let my mother touch him.

———————

The hardest part each morning was trying to brush Mum's teeth. She simply couldn't figure out what to do with the toothbrush. I'd put some toothpaste on the brush and try to show her what I wanted her to do, but after a while it was useless. I had to brush them for her if I wanted them brushed at all.

One of the most difficult and painful behaviour changes carers have to face is the loss of their loved ones' memory of self as they fail to recognize themselves.

One morning my mother was sitting in her rocking chair in the bedroom while I cleaned out a cupboard in the hall. All of a sudden I heard her crying and rushed into the bedroom to see what was the matter. She was looking in the mirror repeating the same phrase over and over again: 'I lost myself. I lost myself.'

No less painful is the realization that our loved ones don't seem to know *us* and may have delusions that we are someone else.

I remember one day my mother said to my Dad, 'She wants me to sit down. Who is she? Do you know who she is?'

If there was anything left of my heart to break, it broke right there. I walked into our back garden and cried my eyes out.

———————

It got to the point that my father didn't recognize my mother. He thought she was a stranger and would lock her out of the house.

If their dog needed to go out at night, my mother

had to go out the kitchen door and onto the porch to let the dog out the porch door. Sometimes Dad would get up and lock the kitchen door behind her, and then he wouldn't let her back in.

Twenty-four hours a day she had to wear a key around her neck.

My wife finally decided I didn't belong to her. I wasn't her husband. I had no business being in the bedroom with her.

She would rant and rave and carry on about the strange man in her room and kept telling me she didn't have to sleep in the same room with a man.

I told her I wouldn't touch her, that I was just there if she needed help, but she said she didn't need me and was perfectly able to take care of herself.

I used to have to wait until she was asleep to go to bed myself. Do you know how that made me feel?

Some people with Alzheimer's retain some recognition of themselves far into the disease but have no idea who others are or where they are. Many continue to live in memories of the past.

Anna Wilcox lived in a nursing home where I worked. She was always certain of her identity, if not the time or the place. If you asked her name, she'd declare with authority and in a very loud voice, 'My name is Anna Wilcox!' But if you asked her if she knew where she was, she'd usually say she was in Ohio, teaching a class of fifteen students in a one-room schoolhouse. The year was somewhere around 1939.

In the evenings when I would tuck her in and turn out her light, she'd tell me about the school. I didn't try to reorientate her to reality. At Anna's stage of dementia, reality orientation usually doesn't work. It only frustrates. So instead I asked her to tell me about the school in Ohio and the children she taught. And she did.

Often it didn't make much sense. She rambled a lot and sometimes mixed up her role as a schoolteacher with her role as a waitress, another job she apparently held for a time. But it really didn't matter at nine o'clock at night. I'd rub her back a little, listen to her stories. Soon she'd be fast asleep with a smile on her face, dreaming, I like to think, about the past.

Simple Memory Joggers

There are many faces of memory loss with Alzheimer's disease. As carers we need to accept and acknowledge them, then help our relatives deal with them one by one, a day at a time, as the disease progresses.

Here are a few suggestions. Some of the initial ideas can be utilized with the loved one who is still living at home in the early stages of the disease. Others can be helpful as the disease progresses and the ability to read and comprehend written instructions is lost.

- A large wall calendar can help a person keep track of time. Hang a pen nearby so the days can be crossed off as they pass.

- Provide a simple list of the day's activities in the order in which they should occur. For example, 1. Eat breakfast. 2. Take green pill with milk. 3. Feed cat.

  Post the list in a conspicuous place.

- Some people with early dementia prefer note cards with memory-jogging information on them about tasks to complete, phone numbers to remember and so on. These can be kept in a small file box with dividers for different subjects.

- If telling time is a problem, consider switching to digital clocks. It may be easier to read the time than to figure it out. This technique completely cured my mother of asking 'What time is it?' literally dozens of times a day, and it greatly relieved her stress and anxiety. We put inexpensive digital clocks in the bedroom, living room and kitchen. For some memory-impaired people, however, the reverse is true: an old-fashioned clock face is easier to read.

- Pill boxes labelled for the day of the week and time of day are available in some chemists. These can be effective in the early stages of Alzheimer's if a sufferer, though still able personally to take medication, might mix up pill bottles. Some people create their own pill boxes with egg boxes. You or a district nurse will need to refill and monitor this system on a regular basis.

- Avoid moving things around in the house. Having things in familiar places is an aid to memory, as is keeping to a familiar routine.

- Pictures and/or labels may help a person identify various rooms in the house. For example, if your relative has trouble finding the bathroom, colour code the door or put a sign on it identifying it. As the disease progresses you may need to switch to a picture of a bath or toilet.

- Some nursing homes have the names or photographs of confused residents outside their rooms. You might also do this in the home. If your loved one can no longer recognize a personal photograph, hang some type of identifying article of clothing such as an old familiar hat or sweater.

My mother began to identify her bedroom when we hung a picture of her grandmother and grandfather next to the door. Prior to that, she kept getting lost.

- Labels on various items in the home—hot and cold water taps and the contents of drawers—can also help jog the memory. Again, as the disease progresses, you might switch from large written labels to pictures of actual drawer contents.

- Let *habit* help you. The person you care for may still be able to perform many routine tasks of daily living with a little help from you. Often the problem lies in initiating the activity. Once it is started, habit seems to take over, and routine tasks can continue to be carried out.

   For example, you may have to put the toothpaste on the brush, hold the brush to your relative's mouth and begin brushing. He or she then may be able to finish the job. Or you may have to cut up food, place some food on a fork and guide hand to mouth a couple of times until the connection is made.

Maintain independence for as long as possible for both your sakes.

Maintaining People Awareness

- Spend time with your loved one reminiscing. Reminiscence or 'life review' is a technique frequently used in nursing homes for older people without dementia. It may also be a helpful intervention for people in the early stages of dementia.

   Talking about people and events from the past, flipping through old photo albums, reading aloud old letters from friends and relatives, looking at old mementos—all of these activities can help maintain some awareness of self and others. They can also serve to draw you and your loved one closer together. Old familiar songs or hymns that have been an important part of his or her life can be used in all stages of the disease. This 'music therapy' can be particularly valuable in the later stages, especially at night.

• Trying to convince people with Alzheimer's that you aren't who they think you are, or that you are who they think you aren't, is probably futile. It may simply provoke a catastrophic or emotional reaction. During nonstressful times, however (and there will be many), remind your loved one of who you are. Say his or her name frequently, too. Our names are important. They're part of our identity. For Alzheimer's sufferers, they can quickly be lost.

• The Alzheimer's sufferer may revert, at various times, to living in the past. As the disease progresses, trying to reorientate to reality may no longer work. A better approach may often be to help your loved one focus attention on events from the past and the feelings associated with them.

We all live in the past to a certain extent. We all spend some time daily remembering various events, both good and bad, that were important to us. These events evoke memories and feelings that make us glad or sad. We might assume that the same happens to our loved ones. Instead of getting upset and trying to orientate them to the present, we need to help them focus on these events. They may need to talk about them and express their feelings.

Thingamajigs and Thingamabobs

Two of my mother's favourite words when I was growing up were *thingamajig* and *thingamabob*. You could always use those words in a pinch if you couldn't remember the name of some-thing. They were handy words. We liked them.

As Mum's disease progressed, virtually everything be-came a 'thingamajig' or 'thingamabob.' It became increas-ingly difficult for her to name familiar objects, to complete sentences and, finally, to communicate any thoughts what-soever.

Language loss as well as memory loss is common in Alzheimer's disease. One frequent behaviour pattern is the substitution of wrong words for right words, especially at the end of a sentence:

> One of the first symptoms we noticed early in the
> progression of my wife's disease was word substitution.
> This continued for a long time. She'd say something
> like 'I need to go out and get the bird' when she meant
> she had to go out and get the post. Or she needed to
> 'cook the car' when she meant she needed to cook
> dinner. I could usually work out what she meant, but
> she certainly confused a lot of other people.

Some people can manage to express a few words of a sentence but not the complete thought. Their communica-tion may sound as if they are reading out of a child's reading book where all the words are nouns and verbs:

> My husband's conversation became short and clipped.
> He'd say 'go' when he wanted to go for a ride, 'eat'
> when he was hungry, and 'love' when he wanted to hug
> or be hugged.

Repetitive or perseverative speech is a frequent problem and, for carers, can be one of the most annoying symptoms of the disease. Words, phrases and questions are often repeated over and over again:

My wife kept repeating herself until I thought I'd go crazy. Sometimes it was the same word. But the worst thing was the same question—'What time is it? What time is it? What time is it?' And I always felt I had to answer her.

Sometimes people with dementia revert to the language of their youth:

In the nursing home my father reverted to his childhood language. His mother came from Czechoslovakia and they always talked the Bohemian language at home. For one period of time, when he was still able to talk, he kept bouncing back and forth between English and Bohemian. It drove the nurses crazy.

The ability to complete sentences may be lost:

My wife would start a sentence. She'd get three or four words out, and the rest was just gibberish. It used to make me feel so bad because I didn't know what she was trying to tell me. She looked so earnest. I would say, 'Is that right?' And that seemed to please her even though it didn't satisfy me.

———————

Once in a while a word comes out I can understand, like 'Christmas,' or a phrase like 'It's cold in here.' But most of the time my husband just babbles. Sometimes we sit and babble together. I love to hear his voice. I dread the day when his babbling stops. Can you understand that?

Eventually language may fail altogether.

Now my father can't even form words to talk to me. It's like his tongue is three times its normal size. He tries to say something once in a while but no intelligible word will come out.

If I say, 'Dad, are you okay?' he may shake his head yes or no. Then again, he may not.

Breaking Through the Walls

Language losses are not easy to deal with, but the following tips may help facilitate both giving and receiving information as you learn new ways to communicate.

- Face your loved one when speaking and maintain eye contact. Speak slowly and distinctly and lower the pitch of your voice. This is especially important if there is any hearing impairment. A low voice is more important than a loud voice.

- Ask questions or give directions one at a time. Don't expect immediate responses. Give the person you care for time to process the information before answering or actively responding. If he or she is trying to respond verbally but is becoming frustrated, help out. You may need to finish a sentence or supply a word. Help to decrease anxiety.

- Tune in to your loved one's body language. Listen to what is being said by facial expressions, body movements, posture and so forth.

   If an Alzheimer's sufferer is trying to communicate something but can't verbally express it, try asking simple questions that can be answered with yes, no or a head movement. If you suspect he or she is in pain, you may have to point to or touch the area you think might be hurting. Ask for a response with a nod of the head, to see if you are correct.

- There are no sure cures for repetitious verbalizations or behaviour, though looking for possible contributing causes is always a first step. For example, 'oh, oh, oh' repeated over and over may be because of pain or the need to go to the toilet.

  Sometimes you can determine no underlying reason for the behaviour, even though your loved one seems anxious and troubled. If you say 'It's okay' or 'It's all right' and show affection, you may help the sufferer feel less anxious and more secure.

  Music may also be helpful for curing repetition. Sarah White, a nursing-home resident diagnosed with Alzheimer's, constantly tapped her foot on the floor and her fingers on the arm of her wheelchair. She also repeated, 'I'm lost, I'm lost, I'm lost.'

  One day we discovered that Sarah had been a minister's wife and a minister's daughter. Church attendance had been a regular part of her life, but no one knew it at the home. So we began taking her to weekly church services. As soon as she heard the music playing and the congregation singing Sarah stopped her repetitious tapping, except to keep time to the music. She also stopped saying, 'I'm lost.'

  We finally got a radio for Sarah's room and kept it tuned to religious or classical music programmes. The music seemed to soothe her, and the repetitious, perseverative behaviour and verbalizations diminished.

  If all your attempts to intervene and break the cycle of repetition fail, you may have to simply remove yourself from the scene for a while to keep from blowing your cool. Pray for patience to weather it until next time.

The many faces of memory loss are indeed painful to see, but the losses can be lessened as we look for ways to preserve and enhance the memory that still exists.

CHAPTER SIX

Emotional Fireworks

We never fought when I was growing up. My mother was very sweet, gentle and easy-going. But we fought when she got Alzheimer's.

One dictionary definition of *catastrophe* is 'a sudden, violent change, such as an earthquake.' This well describes the various catastrophic reactions that frequently accompany Alzheimer's, ranging from the slight tremor of anxiety to a sometimes violent verbal or physical outburst.

Catastrophic reactions are hard to understand. A closer look, however, can often indicate some underlying reasons for our loved one's bizarre behaviour. We need to be aware of the various pressure points that might suddenly trigger an emotional eruption.

Triggers for Catastrophic Reactions

Catastrophic reactions can occur when an Alzheimer's sufferer is frustrated by diminishing abilities:

My dad had been an excellent mechanic. But it got to the point where he ruined everything he touched. It was the most pitiful thing to see.

I'll never forget one experience. Dad's jeep was sitting in the garage and he was tinkering with it, trying to get it to run. He finally came running into the house, absolutely beside himself. 'I can't do it,' he was crying. 'I can't do it. Would you fix my jeep? Would you fix my jeep?'

That broke my heart.

Reactions can sometimes be triggered by irrational fears. They may be accompanied by paranoia.

The district nurse would try to give my husband a bath or even just wash him, and he'd fight. You couldn't struggle with him because you'd lose. He had the strength of a bull. He wouldn't let anyone near him. He'd say that the water was cold, that he was afraid of it.

My mother was absolutely terrified one evening, and she kept pointing to the double door to our patio. I was sure someone was out there, but then I realized she was seeing her own reflection in the glass. I remembered to keep the curtains closed after that episode.

Once, when my mother was still driving, she looked in the rearview mirror and really got hysterical. She was sure the person in the car behind us was following us.

The person in the car was my brother!

Catastrophic reactions can sometimes be triggered by specific actions on the part of another person, especially if the other person is perceived as a threat in any way.

If my father felt threatened he would pinch or hit, especially if you tried to get him to do something he didn't want to.

One night I had to take my mother to the hospital for a medical emergency, and a friend of mine stayed with my father. My father kept wanting to go to the hospital too, and he tried to get in the car. He hit my friend over the head with a torch three times when she tried to stop him.

Reactions can occur when we try to get our loved one to choose among various options or respond to several questions at once:

I remember taking my father to restaurants. I was trying to make him feel better about himself, so I would always ask him to choose what he wanted to eat; I wanted to give him a choice. But instead of feeling better he became frustrated and upset because there were too many things to choose from. He couldn't process all that information, and once he even started to cry. When I finally understood what was happening, we still went out, but I simply ordered for us both.

Catastrophic reactions usually seem like marked personality changes. They are sometimes accompanied by outpourings of profanity and verbal abuse, directed at us. Occasionally they turn into physical violence.

My husband got nasty, really nasty and he was never nasty in his life. He even punched me once with his fists.

One minute my wife seems to know who we are, and five minutes later she'll be yelling and calling us names. It's just as if somebody turns a switch and another person appears. She gets violent and very abusive, just the opposite of what she used to be.

She was one of the most lovable people. There wasn't enough she could do for other people. Not enough. And she never swore. But since she's developed Alzheimer's, I've learned language from her I didn't know existed.

It's a natural tendency to respond to our loved one's catastrophic reactions with emotional outbursts of our own. Catastrophic reactions are stressful and emotionally charged experiences, and if we're feeling unduly stressed to begin with we will react rather than respond. But if we do that, we're in for trouble. As soon as the episode is over, we'll feel like a failure because of the way we handled the situation.

The key phrase to remember when confronted with a catastrophic reaction on the part of a loved one is *keep cool*. That may seem difficult if not impossible to do given the circumstances, but it is the best advice we can give ourselves. It will help to divert disaster and convert catastrophes into experiences we and our loved ones will be able to live through.

What to Do and What to Avoid

The following dos and don'ts offer some practical suggestions.

• Do avoid situations or events which might trigger catastrophic reactions. If you can't avoid them, anticipate them. For example, if you must take your loved one food shopping, avoid Saturday mornings and Friday nights.

Go at times when the supermarket is less likely to be a hive of people. If you go out to eat, avoid the busy hours when restaurants are crowded.

- Do make life as predictable as possible. Most of us get tired of the same old grind, but people with dementia find a daily routine secure and comfortable. Marked schedule changes may precipitate catastrophic reactions. Plan your loved one's life as much as possible. This may become less of a problem as the disease progresses.

- Do limit choices. Remember that your loved one's ability to discriminate is markedly affected by Alzheimer's. If you are helping your mother or wife dress, for example, asking her to choose the blue, brown, yellow or white dress may overwhelm her. You might show her two dresses and ask her to choose one. Or you may simply have to choose one for her.

  Use simple sentences. Offer one thought at a time. Let one task be completed before talking about another one.

- Do simplify the activities of daily living. In the area of clothing, consider substituting pullover dresses, shirts and sweaters for those that button; slip-on loafers for shoes with laces; and Velcro fasteners for zippers, buttons and snaps. Such replacements will help your loved one maintain independence for as long as possible while minimizing catastrophic reactions.

- Don't talk about your loved one's behaviour problems to others in the presence of your loved one. Just because someone may no longer be able to communicate verbally does not mean he or she no longer understands what's going on or what's being said. Think about how you'd feel in a similar situation and be sensitive. Always assume more understanding and comprehension than you actually see.

- Don't take personally the things your loved one says. You or other family members may be accused of stealing money, selling the family home or withdrawing your love. Attempting to deny the accusations may only make things worse.

  If accused of stealing money, for example, you might offer to help search for it. One carer I interviewed has a locked box for which she keeps the key. Inside the box are her mother's cheque-book, recent bank receipts and a little cash. If her mother accuses her of theft, they search for the box together. When they 'find' it, her mother leafs through the bank statements and the cheque-book and usually concludes that all is intact. The catastrophic reaction blows over.

- Don't argue or try to reason. Remember that the disease affects the memory and the mind's ability to think logically. Sufferers may not understand why it isn't safe for them to drive the family car. To believe that they will understand if someone just explains it enough times is an error in judgement. Arguments can also make your loved one more suspicious and defensive, attitude changes you don't need.

  Instead of arguing and reasoning, acknowledge and validate. The disorientation and confusion that are part of Alzheimer's result in more than just bizarre behaviour. Dementia also stirs up deep feelings—for us *and* the people we care for. These feelings seem to have little to do with intellectual impairment. Beneath a belligerent exterior, Alzheimer's sufferers may be nursing a lot of fear, disappointment and hurt, just as we would if we were frustrated in our attempts to do something we'd always loved to do, something that was an important part of our identity. Helping our loved ones to verbalize those feelings, or even to cry, may be the best thing we can do.

- Do avoid shouting or raising your voice. Don't correct or confront the bizarre behaviour. A loud, accusatory voice implies that we somehow expect change in the behaviour. We need to remember that the behaviour is not deliberate. Alzheimer's sufferers don't want to act the way they do.

  Avoid the 'why' questions: 'Why are you doing this?' or 'Why did you do it?' 'Why' questions can put others on the defensive. They feel they have to justify their behaviour, which in this case they're not responsible for. The normal reaction to a perceived threat is fight or flight. Both are catastrophic reactions. What our loved ones need most is our love and acceptance of who they are, just the way they are.

  Speak softly, treating the person you care for with the same dignity and respect you would want to be shown if you were in the same shoes. A proverb in the Bible says, 'A gentle answer quiets anger, but a harsh one stirs it up.' Soothing answers and soft tones can temper many a catastrophic reaction.

- Do move beyond the event and forget it as quickly as possible. Defuse situations by using a technique called distraction. Distraction might include changing the subject, going for a walk to 'search' for the missing item, offering a favourite food to eat.

  Be thankful for your loved one's short-term memory and consider it a blessing in the case of catastrophic reactions.

- Don't physically restrain your relative unless it's absolutely necessary. He or she may feel fenced in and become even more combative.

Instead, capitalize on the excess energy at this time. If your loved one is turning over the living room furniture, it might be an ideal time to clean the carpet! Try to redirect the energy and get him or her to help you.

- Do consider the possibility that medication, such as a mild tranquilizer, may help some people. Catastrophic reactions are often like dormant volcanoes: they suddenly erupt without much warning and are over as quickly as they started. But in some cases the catastrophe may seem continuous. If this is the case for you, talk with your doctor about possible medication.

- Do remove yourself from emotionally charged situations. If you feel you are going to explode, you probably will. It's no sin to walk away if you think the situation is going to get the best of you or if you anticipate physical violence. If you can do so without endangering anyone's safety, leave the scene for a time and return when everyone has calmed down.

- Avoid emotionally distancing yourself. Reach out with a warm embrace, a kiss, a touch of your hand. Affection often can defuse a difficult situation. Touch can communicate that you care. It can offer reassurance and affirmation as well as affection.

'Perfect love drives out fear,' says a verse in the New Testament. Our love for the people we care for may not be perfect. In fact, we may feel very unloving at times. But it will ultimately be love that will drive out the fears we have—and the fears our loved ones have—in dealing with the various catastrophic reactions of Alzheimer's.

Relying on a Greater Power

Sometimes we need to draw on someone other than ourselves, stronger than ourselves, to meet our loved one's needs. This is particularly true in relation to catastrophic reactions.

Several years ago I was working for a home nursing agency when I got a call in the middle of the night from Mrs. Blake, one of our clients. Her husband, who had Alzheimer's, was having a catastrophic reaction. All six feet four inches of him was trying desperately to get out of the house. The only thing standing in his way was his four foot ten inch wife. 'What do I do?' she asked. 'Can you come round?'

My first inclination was to go and help, but I knew that would mean delay. At the time my own mother had a tendency to wander at night. I couldn't leave her alone. Getting her up and dressed to go with me would be a major, time-consuming project.

My second inclination was to call the ambulance or the local police. Surely they'd have the manpower to help this poor woman. But when I mentioned it, she said no, she'd rather not have them there. She wanted to handle it alone.

At that point I was stumped. I told her I'd ring her back in a few minutes and I hung up the phone, thinking through various strategies.

Then I did something I'd done many times before, with my own mother, in similar situations. I prayed. I asked God to give Mrs. Blake wisdom and courage, to protect her and her husband from physical harm, and to defuse that explosive situation.

Five minutes later, I rang back.

'Goodness!' Mrs. Blake said. 'A few minutes after you called, my husband stopped storming around, went over to his chair and sat down. Now he's sleeping like a baby. I guess we'll be okay.'

I guess we'll be okay. Talking to God may not be the first thing that comes to our mind in the middle of a catastrophic reaction, but when we care very much for our loved ones, prayer can remind us that someone else cares too.

CHAPTER SEVEN
Always on the Move

I once worked in a nursing home that had a locked ward. All the residents there had some form of dementia, and all were free to roam and wander around. If the wing had not been locked, many simply would have wandered off—including Sam Smith.

Sam was a man in his eighties. In his younger years he had worked as a guard on the local railway; when Sam stood by the locked door of the ward, he still looked the part. He wore his old battered guard's cap and carried a paper bag filled with biscuits. 'My lunch,' he'd say, if anyone asked. And if anyone questioned why he was waiting by the door the same time every day, Sam would smile and say, 'Waiting for the train.'

When the evening nurses pressed the buzzer on the outside of the door to signal the day staff they had arrived, Sam would get excited. He thought it was the train whistle.

'Not today, Sam. Not today,' the nurses would say as they filed through the door. Tomorrow maybe, but not today.

Sam would continue to pace back and forth by the door for an hour after the shift change. Then he'd go back to his room and wait for tomorrow's train.

Sundowning

When the sun goes down, people with Alzheimer's frequently want to get up and go. Confusion heightens at this time of day. Restless wandering and agitation increase. In the US this phenomenon is called *sundowning*.

Sundowning is a common occurrence in nursing homes. It also occurs at home, and it is often accompanied by catastrophic reactions.

> My wife's restlessness and agitation seem to be worse in the winter months, when the days get shorter and it gets dark early in the afternoon.
>
> Sometimes she gets angry along with getting restless and agitated. Her anger might last half an hour or four or five hours. That big crack in the window over there happened late one afternoon when my wife got angry and threw her shoe.

Reasons for sundowning are unclear, though late-afternoon fatigue may be a contributing factor. It's also wise to consider obvious and correctable physical catalysts for odd behaviour: hunger, thirst or the need to go to the toilet.

If rest, food, drink or elimination fail to calm your loved one's agitation, there are some things you can do to cope with it.

Simplify the environment. In nursing homes, sundowning frequently occurs during shift changes, when nurses and assistants are coming and going and causing confusion. Some times of day are more confusing than others in the home as well. For example, a younger Alzheimer's victim with school-age children may find after-school time particularly stressful. The kids come home with their friends, the television blares, the house is in an uproar.

You may not be able to change the environment, but perhaps you can move your loved one to a room away from busy traffic. Total isolation isn't always necessary, but quieter surroundings may help decrease stress.

If you're able to provide a 'locked ward' type of environment, either in a room of your home or in a fenced area outside, do so. This will enable the person you care for to roam at will and, hopefully, work off some excess energy.

Find simple things for your loved one to do. One helpful idea comes from a carer who calls it a 'rummage box.'

> I made up what I call Mary's rummage box. Every afternoon Mary would enter other people's rooms in our adult home and go through their chests of drawers. Needless to say she wasn't very popular with some of the more alert people.
>
> I got Mary a big box and filled it with soft things like facecloths, towels, balls of wool and soft toys. Then I sat Mary down at the kitchen table while I got dinner ready. For an hour or so she seemed content just taking the things out of the box one by one and putting them back in. She'd also fold and unfold the towels and facecloths.

Spend time with your loved one. Let him or her be near you. Feelings of insecurity may contribute to sundowning. Your loved one may need the reassurance that you, unlike the setting sun, won't leave.

Find easy things to do together that are meaningful and productive: washing up and drying dishes, sweeping the floor, folding laundry, cooking dinner. Even if you have to re-wash, re-sweep, re-fold or re-peel, the fact that you're able to continue sharing in these daily activities is worth the extra time.

An Alzheimer's sufferer may not be able to clean the whole house or cook an entire meal, but the loss of these abilities is usually gradual. You can capitalize on the abilities that are still intact and help preserve them for as long as possible. When you do that, you also help preserve your loved one's self-esteem.

If your relative is manageable, perhaps late afternoon is the best time to shop for food, do errands or simply get away from it all. Go for a drive and enjoy the scenery together.

Reliving pleasures from the past may also be a means of calming down a person with Alzheimer's. Consider watching an old film on television, looking through photo albums and talking about old times, old friends. Sing some favourite songs or hymns. Put on a record and dance. Do what you used to do. Focus on the familiar.

Late afternoon may also be a good time to take a walk. It's good exercise for you both, and you might find that a late-afternoon exercise break will decrease nightly wandering and enhance your relative's ability to sleep.

Sundowning can indeed cause frustration and anxiety for everyone in the family touched by Alzheimer's disease. But it can also be an incentive for new dimensions of creativity and companionship.

Prone to Wander

You'd think a lot of restless wandering throughout the day would exhaust your loved one as much as it does you, but this is not always the case. Many people with Alzheimer's continue to wander well into the night and on into the early hours of the morning.

> I was always on the alert. My husband would get up around 2:00 a.m. and turn on the light in our room.
> He'd pack a suitcase, or sometimes just a box of

trinkets, and head downstairs. Sometimes he'd just roll his bedding up and take it downstairs and pile it on the floor. Usually he got dressed.

So then I'd get out of my bed and put my dressing gown on and go downstairs with him, and we'd just sit in the living room chairs in the dark until 4:00 or 5:00 a.m. and then we'd both go back to bed for a while.

He never tried to go out at night, but he was up for most of it.

———————————

My wife started living in the past, living on the farm where she grew up. She was always getting out of bed in the middle of the night. Then she'd wander all through the house, looking for the animals.

———————————

My husband wandered all over the house at night. I stayed awake to make sure he was all right.

The doctor wanted me to tie my husband in bed so I could get some rest, but I just couldn't. And the medications he gave him only seemed to make him worse—especially during the day.

So he wandered and I didn't get much sleep. I finally hired people to stay at night, but that first year was terrible.

If wandering around the house at night is part of your relative's lifestyle, the following suggestions may be helpful. As always with behaviour management problems, think about physical causes first.

Hunger or thirst can contribute to restless wandering. Your loved one may be looking for food. Offer a small glass of warm milk or herbal tea just before retiring. Avoid anything with caffeine, including hot chocolate. Consider the addition of complex carbohydrate foods, such as a sandwich or biscuits and cheese.

On the other hand, what you perceive as restlessness may be the sign of a full bladder. Be sure there is a visit to the toilet before retiring, and watch out for excessive fluid intake for several hours prior to going to bed. You might also try placing a commode in a strategic spot, either at the foot of the bed or in front of the bedroom door if finding the bathroom in the middle of the night presents a problem.

If your relative suffers from some other malady in addition to Alzheimer's that may cause pain, consider appropriate pain medication at night. Pain can contribute to agitation.

Nightly wandering may be a symptom of daily inertia. What may be needed during daylight hours is some sort of sustained activity such as a planned walk or two around the block.

Think about the effect environmental cues might have on confused people. If the person you care for gets up at night and spots his coat and hat on the chair and his clothes all neatly laid out for the next morning, he may assume it already *is* the next morning, get up and get dressed. You also might want to disguise obvious exits with not-so-obvious curtains.

A warm bath or shower prior to retiring may help your loved one relax. Avoid bubble baths. They can contribute to urinary tract infections, a complication you don't need. Follow the bath with a soothing back rub.

Keep a bedside radio tuned softly to a classical-music station or to the type of music your loved one has always enjoyed. Some carers leave the television turned on low. Experiment if necessary. A chat show may be the perfect soporific.

Many people have been used to reading a book before

retiring. Reading to your loved one from a familiar source may help induce sleep.

Cuddly things can be comforting and seem to lend a sense of security. Many nursing homes encourage families to bring in soft toys. This can also work in the home for some people.

Sleep medication may be the answer for some, but it should generally be used as a last resort. You will need a prescription for most medications. You might ask your doctor for a dosage range and be sure the medication is in a low-enough dose to allow you to experiment. Never use more when less will do. If tranquilizers are taken during the day, you might be able to divide them up so the stronger dose can be given at night.

Remember that all medications, including sleep medications, have side effects. A medication that one person tolerates well can send another person into a tailspin. This is true for over-the-counter sleep medications as well as prescription drugs. Some may even stimulate rather than depress the central nervous system.

Vest or waist restraints may help but should be used cautiously. Some people adjust to them well; others fight them. Request assistance from your district nurse to attach them in the correct way to the patient and to the bed. They need to be tied securely enough so your loved one won't escape and fall. Make certain you can untie them quickly in case of an emergency. There are a variety of styles to choose from.

Consider hiring a private nurse or carer for the night shift to allow you to get some sleep. Use the skills of the substitute carers you hire. Remember, you are paying them. They shouldn't be sleeping on the job!

Set up a plan with them or their agency that will include their responsibilities, for example, a morning routine of bathing, toileting, dressing, shaving, nail care, and so on.

Let them do the tasks you find difficult to do or that rob you of your needed energy. If your loved one is awake for large blocks of time in the night, some of these activities could be completed then, while you sleep.

Be aware that some people with Alzheimer's may get up, get dressed, wander around the house for an hour or so, then head for the nearest chair or sofa and promptly fall asleep. Don't worry too much about where they sleep or what they're wearing. The important thing is that they do sleep.

If, in spite of all your efforts, the person you're caring for is still prone to wander nocturnally, you'll need to provide for safety. See Chapter Nine for more information about this subject.

Leaving Home

Bill Stewart looked out of the kitchen door. The moon hung full, illuminating the path to the road. Helen, Bill's wife, was asleep. She'd locked the kitchen door, just as she always did, but tonight she'd forgotten to remove the key. Bill saw it, turned it and then stepped out into the moonlight.

The town was seven miles north of their farm. Bill turned right at the gate and headed down the lonely country road.

The next morning a frantic Helen and two policemen found Bill curled up on a bench in the centre of town. Sleeping.

Helen and Bill were certainly not alone in their nocturnal experience. People with Alzheimer's frequently wander aimlessly through their homes. Often they wander away from them. Night or day.

Of all the bizarre behaviour patterns of Alzheimer's sufferers, wandering away from home and getting lost is one of the most disturbing to carers.

My husband ran away from home several times. I remember one time when he said he was going to pick blackberries. He took his basket and ran off into the rain. My daughter and I went after him, but we lost him in the woods and had to go back home and call the police.

After we called, we started searching again. We finally found him ourselves, up on the hill. He was soaking wet. And his basket was empty.

———————————

Do you see those geraniums there in the window? Well, one time when I came home from work my wife had taken off. I found a couple of cuttings of geraniums along the street and then I found more. I just kept picking up geranium cuttings until I found her. When we got home I put all the cuttings in water. The ones in the window here are their descendants.

———————————

There were two places I usually thought to look for my wife. One was the church. The other was the supermarket. One day she wasn't at either of those places. I looked everywhere and finally I came home.

After I'd been home awhile I got a phone call from my neighbour. He said he'd seen my wife wandering around a car park, and he'd persuaded her to let him bring her home.

When she was well she would never walk away like that. I don't know where she thought she was going. That car park is three miles away.

———————————

One day Dad ran off into the woods. I spent an hour and a half looking for him. I was about to call the police when he came out of the woods by our neighbour's house, and they called me.

You know, the feelings of guilt and embarrassment we suffered in the beginning were totally unnecessary. But we didn't know what was happening.

Finally I said to my mother, 'This man is sick. It's nothing to be ashamed of. Let's tell everybody.' So we started with the neighbours. I told them all, 'If you see my father wandering, let me know immediately.'

It was a good thing we did that.

Wandering off is not confined to wandering away from home. Sometimes people with Alzheimer's wander away when they're on holiday.

Three years ago my family was at a museum up north. In this museum you had to go in and out of different rooms to see the different exhibits.

We'd gone about two-thirds of the way round when we suddenly realized my wife wasn't with us. We thought she must have come out of one of the rooms and turned in the opposite direction from the rest of us.

We searched. We went all around the building and into other buildings. We looked everywhere. Finally we went out into the car park, and there she was. She'd got into the exit queue and wandered out of the gate.

When we came up to her she said to us, 'Well, I found the car, but I couldn't find the keys. If I had found them I'd have gone home.'

And I think she would have. Or tried to.

That was our first experience of wandering off. There have been many more since.

If your loved one wanders away, you are faced with an emergency situation that could easily turn to tragedy. The phrase to remember is *don't panic*. The following strategies can help you cope:

- Don't spend time blaming yourself for your loved one's disappearance. Guilt won't help find anyone. If needed, call for assistance. Contact neighbours, friends, relatives and the police to aid in the search. It's also good to let other people in the area know your relative is lost. They may not be officially part of the search party, but they can be on the alert. Think about the obvious places your loved one might go—especially places familiar in the past—and share your information with the searchers.

- Search parties need a description of the person they're looking for. Have some recent colour photographs at home. Also keep pictures of your relative in the glove compartment of your car.

- Notify area hospital accident and emergency departments and nursing homes of your loved one's disappearance. If some good Samaritan finds your relative wandering down the road, they might have taken him or her to one of these places.

- Your loved one should have an identification bracelet or necklace that says 'memory impaired,' 'memory loss' or 'Alzheimer's disease.' It can also include name, address and your phone number. If the person has a medical condition in addition to Alzheimer's, such as angina or diabetes, that information should be included along with allergies to any medications. Identification (ID) jewellery can be purchased through some jewellers and inexpensively engraved for you. There's a wide range of prices. Wallet-size ID cards are usually not a good substitute for an ID bracelet or necklace, because they can be easily lost or thrown away.

- Finding your loved one is only half the battle. Now you have to get him or her home.

Chances are that your relative will be relieved to see you. She may be upset and know she's lost. On the other hand, you may not be seen as a rescuer but as someone to fend off or hide from.

Whatever the case, stay calm. Avoid running up, pulling on a sleeve or trying to reason. Remind other rescuers that these techniques probably won't work. Instead, you might ask your loved one where he's going and offer to walk with him or take him with you. Most wanderers are looking for home. Home with you is where they really want to be.

If the person you care for is always on the move, don't despair. With foresight, planning and some practical strategies, we can maintain a relatively safe and secure environment for the perpetual or nocturnal wanderer.

Looking for lost loved ones is a challenge most of us have to face at some point. It's a challenge we will meet when that point comes.

CHAPTER EIGHT

Baffling Behaviour

My mother used to take me visiting with her often when I was a child. Occasionally we'd go to the homes of relatives who had knick-knacks and glassware lying around on tables and shelves, just waiting to be knocked off. But my mother had trained me well. I always walked around with my hands either behind my back or in my pockets. So did she!

When Mum developed Alzheimer's, she acted just the opposite, reaching out and touching everything in sight. Sometimes she took the things she touched.

Hoarding

When I used to go food shopping, Mum usually went with me. I would push her ahead of me in her portable wheelchair and pull the shopping trolley behind us. When our shopping was completed, I carefully checked her pockets and the sleeves of her cardigan before paying. Mum had a tendency, often when I was busy looking in a particular section, to reach out and touch the assortment of packaged cakes and biscuits in the middle of the aisle. If a packet was small, colourful and looked good to eat, my mother might pocket it for future consumption.

In a nursing home where I occasionally work, one

resident has a habit of wandering into other people's rooms and rummaging through their drawers, collecting things to 'take home.' I sometimes find her exiting a room carrying a shoe, a box of paper hankies or underwear.

Asking her to give these items up is like asking a toddler to relinquish a favourite toy. 'No' is always the answer, accompanied by a set jaw and an even firmer grip on the pilfered items. I'm usually able to retrieve them, though, if I offer to swap. The swap might take the form of a biscuit, a glass of milk, or a magazine. Sometimes it takes several exchanges to accomplish the task, but it works and we both wind up happy. (I find this also works with another resident who has a habit of pinching the fire extinguisher!)

People with Alzheimer's are a little like pirates. In the words of Janet Sawyer of the Blumenthal Jewish Home, Clemmons, North Carolina, they love to 'rummage, pillage and hoard.' Then they may pocket the loot (food, shoes, neckties, jewellery, and so forth) and stash it away in a hiding place that they alone seem to know.

It got to the point where everybody was 'stealing' Dad's stuff. He thought people were coming in the house and hiding things from him, but he was really the one who was doing the hiding.

My father was for ever losing his tool-box. It was his prized possession, so he would hide it—and then forget where he hid it. One of his favourite hiding places was under the china cupboard in the living room. But sometimes the tool-box wound up under the bed or down in the cellar.

He'd say to my mother, 'Where are my tools? What did you do with them?' And, to keep the peace, my mother would have to go with him and search for them.

> There was this terrible odour coming from my
> mother's room. The auxiliaries finally worked it out.
> Mum had tucked away a chicken leg in the drawer of
> her bedside table.

How do we solve the problem of taking and losing things?
Asking 'Where did you hide it this time?' never works, but
there are some gentle, loving and practical ways to discover
where your wife stashed the family jewels or your father hid
the house keys.

- Have a place only you know about to put car keys, cash
  and other irreplaceable items. Make small and easily lost
  articles more visible by attaching them to larger and more
  colourful things, like key rings. Try to have duplicates of
  whatever can be duplicated.

- Put bills and other important papers out of reach and out
  of sight. Many Alzheimer's sufferers don't just hide
  things, they also tear them up.

- Check the contents of wastebaskets before throwing out
  the rubbish.

- Lock the toilet door if your loved one has a tendency to
  flush away valuables.

- You may need to lock inner doors, cupboards and
  drawers. This not only protects other people's valuables
  but also eliminates hiding places.

- Think of some of the not-so-obvious places where your
  loved one might hide things, if you're truly stumped.
  Check the folds of chairs and sofas. Examine handbags
  or wallets. Look in bowls and dishes in the kitchen.

- If your relative tends to hoard valuable things, use substitutes. Buy some cheap costume jewellery and store your good stuff in a place your loved one isn't likely to look. If he or she stashes away food that spoils, make packages of savoury biscuits available. Nibbling at various times during the day or night may be the result of legitimate hunger. Provide for this need.

- Keep a 'rummage box' that can be used as a substitute when your loved one starts rummaging through chests or drawers.

- Don't expect your relative to remember the hiding places of the car keys or the post. Asking or demanding will only create a stressful situation. Simply expect to join in the search from time to time.

Rummaging, pillaging, hiding and hoarding are behaviours common to people with Alzheimer's. The reasons are unclear, but the need for security may be an underlying factor. Creating a secure environment is a challenge we all face as we care for our loved ones. It is a challenge that can try our patience. It can also make us more tolerant and sensitive people.

Losing Control

Difficulties with bladder and bowel elimination usually become a problem as Alzheimer's progresses. Incontinence of urine and stool occurs frequently and can present a real physical and emotional dilemma for the unprepared carer. Incontinence can also be embarrassing. It requires us to keep our sense of humour and sense of perspective.

I remember the day my wife had a bowel movement in

the supermarket. I was mortified. But they were so good to us. One young shop assistant came up behind us and rolled up the rug. Luckily my wife did it in the right spot.

My mother was incontinent once right in the bank. I was cashing a cheque and when I turned around, there she was, taking off her wet pants over by the window. I ran over, grabbed the pants, stuffed them in my handbag and got her out of there. Fast.

Just last week I saw a two year old in a shop downtown do the same thing. Her mother reacted the same way I did. I think you need a sense of humour in this business.

My husband is totally incontinent now and has been for quite a while. His urologist told me that one of the things I could expect eventually was lack of control of bowels and bladder. The bad thing about it was that my husband sometimes went to the back of the barn and shed his clothes, including his incontinence pads. He'd throw the wet or soiled pads aside and then put his clothes back on. I think there's quite a pile of those pads out at the back of the barn, in the raspberry bushes.

In addition to getting rid of our embarrassment, we need to lose the notion that toileting is a very personal, very private affair. Sooner or later we may have to get involved in this aspect of our loved one's care.

The biggest problem I had was when my wife first became incontinent. She'd wet the bed at night and I

116

decided, well, I'll just have to get her up. It was tough because she was a sound sleeper and resisted me. Often before I could get her to the toilet she'd urinate on the floor. It used to make me so cross because I didn't understand what was happening.

Finally I decided there was just no sense trying to get her up and getting angry. It didn't do her any good and it didn't do me any good. So I got some disposable adult nappies, a rubber sheet, and some smaller sheets they call draw sheets, and I put them on the bed. If she was swimming in the morning, that was all right. I just had extra laundry to do.

The following are suggestions for preventing and dealing with incontinence, should it occur, as well as other aspects of bladder and bowel management.

- If incontinence of urine becomes a problem at any stage of Alzheimer's disease, don't assume it's due to the Alzheimer's process. This is especially true if symptoms appear suddenly. There may be an underlying medical problem, such as a urinary-tract infection (UTI). Initially it's wise to talk to your doctor. A simple urine test may be recommended to see if there's an infection that could easily be treated with an antibiotic. Untreated urinary-tract infections can worsen any incontinence related to Alzheimer's.

  Women are more prone than men to develop UTIs because it is easier for infectious agents to move up and into the female bladder.

  Symptoms of urinary-tract infections and more severe kidney infections can include any or all of the following:

  frequent urge to urinate
  urinating in small amounts
  difficulty starting to urinate

burning, pain or stinging on urination
foul-smelling urine
cloudy, blood-tinged or mucus-containing urine
abdominal pain or discomfort
fever and chills
nausea and vomiting
back pain
increased confusion

- Some medications can contribute to urinary incontinence: 'water pills' or diuretics, for example. It's usually best to give these early in the morning to prevent incontinence at night.

  Some tranquilizers and sedatives can have the opposite effect and result in urine retention that, if unnoticed and untreated, can be a serious, even life-threatening problem. The medications Haldol or Serenace (both containing haloperidol), frequently prescribed for people with Alzheimer's, are notable examples. Your chemist is usually a good source of information about drug side effects.

  If our loved ones are on medication that can cause urinary side effects we need to carefully observe their toileting habits.

- Anticipate accidents. Become aware of mannerisms that may indicate a need to urinate or have a bowel movement.

- Minimize accidents by having a susceptible person cut down on fluid intake, especially tea and coffee, several hours before bedtime.

  Fluids should not usually be limited during the day, however, except for other medical reasons. Adequate fluid intake is essential for proper hydration and can also help prevent urinary-tract infections and constipation. If in doubt, check with your doctor. The necessary amount of fluid may vary from person to person. Dehydration as well as overhydration can contribute to confusion.

- Toilet at regular intervals—every two to three hours, before or after meals, just prior to retiring. Do this even if your loved one wears an incontinence pad or pants. Through regular toileting, a habit pattern can form that may keep him or her dry throughout the day and night. It's definitely worth your effort and a little trial and error.

- Minimize the distance from bedroom to bathroom. Consider the use of a bedside commode.

- Think about using an adult nappy or pad or, for minimal incontinence and dribbling, a sanitary towel or baby's nappy worn inside the underwear. There are many different brands of pants available through chemists and mail order. Costs vary, and it is worth finding out first what is available from the community nursing services. Some people's skin may be sensitive to some makes. You may need to experiment if your relative develops a rash.

  Ask your district nurse or Continence Adviser for tips on how to put the adult 'nappies' on when a person is lying down or standing up. Rubber pants are also available in adult sizes.

  Protective pads may help your loved one (and you) feel more secure when out and about, though there is often an understandable initial reaction to 'needing to wear nappies again, like a baby', as one carer put it. If your relative does not take them off at night, incontinence pads may help you both get a good night's rest. Be sensitive, though, to your loved one's feelings of shame, embarrassment and loss of self-esteem.

- Skin tissue is very sensitive to urine and can break down quickly if not kept clean and dry. Soap and water is all you need. Avoid perfumed powders: they can contribute to urinary-tract infections. Cornflour may be an alternative if perspiration around skin folds in the abdomen and groin area is a problem.

  As with urine, stool on the skin can result in skin breakdown and even urinary-tract infections. If you need to assist your loved one with hygiene, wipe and wash well, wiping and/or washing from front (urinary opening) to back (rectal area).

- Protect the bed with a waterproof mattress cover. A large sheet of plastic or an old shower curtain also works well. Disposable or cloth bed pads with waterproof backing are available and can cut down on laundry. Simple draw sheets (smaller pieces of sheeting) or pillowcases with a piece of plastic inside may also work well and are inexpensive alternatives.

  To control odours from urine, wash mattress covers regularly with soap and water, and disinfectant.

  Some areas have an incontinence laundry service which can be a great help for carers. It is worth asking your district nurse whether such a service is available.

- Indwelling catheters are usually not recommended for the management of incontinence because they can easily contribute to infections and are often pulled out by people with dementia. External catheters that fit like condoms may, however, be useful for some men who experience incontinence at night and are heavy sleepers.

- If urinary retention and difficulty starting a urine stream are problems, try running water in the sink or bath when your loved one is on the toilet.

Your GP should be able to provide information on how to contact a local Continence Adviser for further help.

Bowel habits differ from person to person. Some people move their bowels daily, others every two to three days. A person with dementia may have difficulty keeping a normal schedule for a variety of reasons related to the disease process, diet, lack of exercise, various medications, and so on. If diarrhoea is a problem, it may be related to a stomach upset or injudicious use of laxatives.

A more frequently occurring problem is constipation. Signs of constipation include pain in the abdominal or rectal area, irregular and infrequent bowel movements, discomfort or pain when having a bowel movement, diarrhoea or liquid leakage around a hard, impacted stool, headache.

The best way to prevent constipation is through a diet adequate in liquids, fibre and bulk. Breakfast is often the best meal for adding fibre. You might try sprinkling bran on hot cereal or serving a high-fibre cereal. (A fibre cereal mixed with yogurt and fruit is a nutritious way to increase fibre and bulk.) Substitute wholemeal breads for white. Generally add more raw fruits and vegetables to the menu of the person you care for.

● Lack of exercise can contribute to constipation. Remember the therapeutic value of walking.

● Constipation is also a frequent side effect of some medications, especially those prescribed for pain. Ask your chemist. You may need to switch to another type of pain reliever if the problem persists.

● If diet and exercise fail to work, consider the use of stool softeners, either prescription or over-the-counter. Some are available in liquid or powder form. Overuse of laxatives such as milk of magnesia may lead to bowel inactivity. Avoid them, if possible.

- Suppositories may help some people. They are available in mild over-the-counter forms or by prescription. Chemists also carry various brands of enema that are relatively easy to administer and may need to be used on occasion. If you have any questions about how to give an enema, check with your district nurse.

Losing control can be an embarrassment for the Alzheimer's sufferer and a management problem for the carer. But we need to remember that it is a *manageable* problem, a problem that can be minimized with the proper resources and our resourcefulness.

Managing Mealtimes

Mealtimes usually include fun and fellowship as well as food. But when you're caring for a person with Alzheimer's, mealtimes can be times of frustration.

Eating isn't always a sit-down occasion:

> My father wouldn't sit down for his meals. He decided he'd rather stand. He'd say, 'I gotta do this' and 'I gotta do that,' and then he'd eat a little and run around the house. He was extremely hyperactive. Extremely.

Judgment and co-ordination are sometimes affected:

> My brother can't always judge where his food is. We have to put it in his hand. He does a lot better with finger food, with things he can feel. Cutlery seems too hard for him to manage, and I think he has trouble

feeling it because it's so thin. He eats sandwiches, bananas, cheese, things like that.

The memory for eating and perhaps even for swallowing becomes impaired for some people:

My mother sits down at the table but then can't remember how to eat, what to do with her fork or spoon. I usually have to get her started, and then sometimes the old memory seems to come back and kick in. At other times it doesn't, and I have to feed her an entire meal.

It got so it took for ever for my wife to eat. It took over an hour for lunch. Sometimes she'd chew something for ten minutes before she'd swallow it.

You know how you might stroke a baby's throat? That's what I'd do with my wife. I'd say, 'Come on, now. Swallow, swallow, swallow.' And then, when she was ready, she'd swallow.

Sometimes a person may refuse to eat. At other times he or she will eat everything in sight:

My husband eats everything he can get his hands on, but he doesn't gain any weight. He runs it off the rest of the time.

My wife seemed to lose her appetite one day and refused to eat. Now it's a hard job to get anything down her. I know she's depressed, too, and that accounts for some of it.

People with Alzheimer's, particularly in the later stages, are prone to respiratory infections like pneumonia. These may be precipitated by choking on and inhaling food.

> Some people with Alzheimer's have trouble swallowing, and then they choke. Instead of food going down their oesophagus it goes down their windpipe. I think that's what happened to my wife. She got pneumonia after an episode of choking one day at the nursing home.

The following suggestions may help make mealtimes more manageable at various stages in the disease:

- Decrease stimulation in the environment. Maintain a calm atmosphere at mealtimes. Play quiet music instead of loud television programmes. Consider subdued lighting instead of a bright glare.

- In meal planning, choose from the basic four food groups for a well-rounded diet. These include for a day:
    Protein. Two to three servings of the following: meat, poultry, fish, cheese, eggs, dried beans, peas, nuts.
    Carbohydrates. Four servings of bread, cereal, potatoes. Wholemeal breads are best.
    Dairy. Two or more servings of milk or milk products such as ice cream, cottage cheese, yogurt.
    Fruits and vegetables. Four or more servings including dark green or deep yellow vegetables, tomatoes and citrus fruits.
    Focus on familiar foods your loved one has always liked. Many finger foods including sandwiches, cheese, fruits and vegetables can meet the 'basic four' requirements and also meet the needs of a person who is always on the go.

- Small, frequent meals or snacks may be more acceptable than large, sit-down dinners three times a day.

- To increase nutrition for the finicky eater, leave snacks around or add the following supplements during the day:
  milk shakes (add ice cream, sweetener, flavouring, an egg to a glass of milk)
  puddings, custards, yogurt
  Complan, Build Up or other diet supplements

- If swallowing or chewing becomes a problem, try grinding or blending foods. This is preferable to tinned baby foods and enables you to cook the same meal for the whole family. A food processor, blender or small grinder will work well. Thick liquids are often swallowed more easily than thinner liquids. Try cream soups for easier swallowing and added nourishment.

- Try the following steps for alleviating co-ordination problems.

  Substitute bowls for plates, or consider using a plate guard to minimize accidental spilling.
  Switch to unbreakable dishes.
  Build up cutlery handles to make them easier to feel and hold.
  Offer only one food at a time if your loved one has difficulty making choices.

- If you must feed your loved one, consider the following.

  Sit, don't stand, when feeding. Maintain eye contact.
  Converse naturally, but don't encourage a lot of talking or laughter that could contribute to choking.
  Spoons often work better than forks for feeding.

Approach your relative directly, not from the side.
Feed using a gentle, downward pressure on the
centre of the tongue.

If there is any weakness or paralysis related to a stroke
or multi-infarct dementia, feed on the unaffected
side to make chewing and swallowing easier.

Be sensitive to the temperature of foods, especially
when foods are microwaved. A person with
dementia may not be able to communicate
discomfort.

Take your time. Don't rush. You may need to encourage your relative to swallow after each bite or make
sure food isn't being squirreled away in bulging
cheeks.

- As an added safety precaution, learn the Heimlich or
abdominal-thrust manoeuvre, a relatively simple procedure that has saved thousands of lives. It is something all
of us should know, with or without a loved one with
Alzheimer's. Hospitals and some nursing homes teach
their employees this procedure. You might be able to ask
your district nurse to teach you or attend a class with St
John's Ambulance. If you can't attend a class or demonstration, refer to a first-aid book.

- Remember that going out to eat doesn't have to stop when
your loved one has Alzheimer's.

I used to take my wife to a luncheon club run by the
community centre in our town. It was good for us both.
It got me out and provided her with more stimulation
than she had at home. We made a lot of friends there too.

I take my husband out to eat quite a lot. He sometimes

spills things, and occasionally I have to feed him. I have a couple of places that we go to pretty regularly, usually when it's not very crowded. They all know us and the waitresses are great. You don't have to stop doing things you've always enjoyed just because you have Alzheimer's, you know.

You *don't* have to stop doing things you've always enjoyed. And enjoying a meal with a loved one at home or away is one of those things that can still be a part of life.

Sexual Disinhibitions

My husband undresses himself a lot in the nursing home, right in the middle of the dining room. Sometimes he asks the other residents and even the aides if they will go to bed with him. If he were in his right mind he'd be humiliated.

My sister was always a very shy, withdrawn person but she isn't anymore. You should hear the language that comes out of her mouth when they try to give her a shower. She also tries to grab people if they get too close to her—and not in very acceptable places.

Loss of impulse control, causing a person to engage in inappropriate sexual behaviour of which they are not aware because of their state of disorientation, is not common to most Alzheimer's sufferers. But when it does occur it can be particularly distressing to the family caregiver at home. If their loved one is in a nursing care facility, family members need to know their loved one will be treated with dignity and respect and not made fun of or treated with contempt.

Often behaviour that may appear sexual in nature may be

caused for various other reasons. For example, the person who wanders around partially clothed or with a blouse unbuttoned or trousers unzipped may have simply forgotten how to dress themselves. Due to the degree of their dementia, they may be totally unaware of their state of undress.

A calm, gentle, but firm approach to reorient a person back to their bedroom or a bathroom where you can assist them in redressing is often all that is needed to solve the problem. In nursing homes, trying to redress a person in a busy hall or noisy dining area will often precipitate a catastrophic reaction. The person may think they are being molested; not a few persons with Alzheimer's have cried 'rape' when caregivers with good intentions have tried to help them.

If zippers on trousers are continually becoming unzipped and shirts and blouses unbuttoned, switch to pull-on trousers and pull-over shirts and sweaters. Dresses that zip in the back are better for women who have a tendency to fidget with their clothes.

Masturbation may also occur in public places and may be engaged in simply because it feels good to the brain-damaged person. Distraction will often work if the person's attention can be redirected to something else to hold or touch. Masturbation can also be prompted by poor genital hygiene, or itching related to a urinary tract infection that prompts rubbing the genital area for relief. Carefully assess possible underlying physical reasons for this behaviour, such as the adequacy of hygiene.

Sexual overtures, or what are interpreted as sexual overtures, may be made in nursing home or hospital settings to other residents, patients, visitors, and staff members. Often the person with dementia will simply mistake the other person for a beloved spouse and treat them accordingly. They may climb into bed with another resident of the opposite sex, simply because they have always slept with a spouse and have no idea that this is not their own room or their own bed. A gentle but firm approach can guide the person with dementia back to their own room and bed; the rights of other residents need to be protected, but the affectional and relationship needs for closeness and companionship of the person with dementia should also be addressed.

The impact of Alzheimer's on the marital relationship, including all the varying dimensions of sexuality and intimacy, can be devastating for caregivers. As Lore Wright, in *Alzheimer's Disease and Marriage* notes, Robert Browning's poem that includes the familiar lines, 'Grow old along with me! The best is yet to be...' rings hollow for many couples when a spouse has Alzheimer's.

Sensitive marital counselling with a professional very familiar with Alzheimer's disease may be needed. Other caregiving spouses can also be supportive and may welcome the opportunity to share concerns and strategies with others in similar situations.

CHAPTER NINE

The Struggle for Safety

Safety is always an issue with older people, especially those living alone and in frail health. Add dementia, and safety becomes an all-consuming concern where neglect can spell catastrophe. Preventive measures have to be taken. And fortunately there are many things we can do to ensure our loved ones' safety, as well as our own.

Taking Away the Car Keys

Most of us drive by habit. If the way is familiar, we're often unaware of the various roads we pass or the towns we drive through. Yet if the sudden and unexpected should occur, all our senses go on the alert. We are usually able to make a quick judgement, respond appropriately and avoid an accident.

This may not be the case, though, with Alzheimer's sufferers, who may be unable to respond quickly or logically to a sudden, unexpected event. Although vision may remain intact and hearing unaffected, the ability to make decisions about what they are seeing and hearing—and even where they are going—is progressively impaired.

One day my husband turned around, right in the middle of the road. We were on the main street in the city at the time. The next thing I knew, we were heading up the slip road—going the wrong way—on to the motorway.

I said to myself, 'This is it. I can't cope with this any longer.'

I used to pray every day for other drivers because my father was a maniac on the road. He had been an excellent mechanic and driver, but as his disease progressed he became careless and dangerous. He gave me a lift one day that was enough to make my hair turn white. It was the most awful experience of my life.

Our identity is partly defined for us by the things we do, particularly the things we do well. Driving is something most of us, especially men, are expected to do and do well.

Being told you cannot drive, that you are no longer safe on the road, can be a tremendous blow to a person's ego. Regardless of the degree of memory impairment, a person still responds on a feeling level when identity is threatened. People with Alzheimer's often won't relinquish the wheel voluntarily.

My husband's driving drove me crazy, but I couldn't convince him to stop. You'd think he'd been on a ten-day drinking binge the way he acted behind the wheel.

I'd shout, I'd scream, I'd stamp my feet. I even threatened to leave him once. It didn't make any difference. He kept insisting he could drive just fine.

My car was being fixed the day we had our family reunion. After the reunion Dad took me to the garage and he started following a motorcycle driver. He was only about two feet ahead of us and the poor guy couldn't go any faster. He was behind another car, sandwiched in by my father.

I said to Dad, 'Don't you think you're a little close?' He just glared at me and said, 'Oh, it's all right.'

He could never understand that his judgement was wrong.

Convincing a loved one to stop driving may be the most difficult thing we'll ever have to do as carers. But it must be done: usually the sooner, the better.

How soon is *soon?* We can take our cues from our loved ones. If there are obvious impairments in other areas that involve judgement, concentration and co-ordination, as well as time, place and person orientation, the ability to drive safely also will be impaired. It will only worsen.

The following strategies may be helpful:

Begin with a gentle person-to-person approach. You may find yourself pleasantly surprised. Your relative may consider it a *relief* not to have to drive. Don't assume he or she wants to continue driving.

Many carers find that it helps to think and pray before talking with the loved one. Avoid judging or criticizing driving skills. Instead, consider the person's feelings and empathize. It should be easy: you know how you'd feel if you were in a similar position. Focus on the safety issues involved.

One carer told me, 'I hid my husband's glasses. I hid the car keys. I removed the distributor cap. I disconnected the starter wire. Alzheimer's makes you really sneaky.'

You may have to do any or all of these things at some point if your loved one insists on driving, though perhaps a

better solution is to visibly remove the object of the tempta-
tion. If you don't drive, this shouldn't be a problem. If you
do, check with a neighbour or nearby garage about keeping
your vehicle for your use only.

Ask your GP to speak with your loved one or write a letter
or a 'prescription' stating he or she can no longer drive.

> The doctor helped me out and it worked just fine. He
> took my husband into his surgery, sat him down and
> said, 'George, how many years have you been driving?
> Don't you think it would be a good idea if you sat in the
> passenger seat for a while and let your wife do the
> driving for you both?'
> I guess it must have been the voice of authority. I
> never had to speak to my husband again. He just quit
> driving.

> My father was always a respecter of the law regarding his
> driving licence. He knew you couldn't drive the car
> without it. He would always say, 'Have I got my licence?'
> We finally convinced the doctor that Dad was dan-
> gerous on the road. The doctor wrote him a letter
> stating he could no longer drive. When we got the
> letter, my dad gave my mother his licence. He just
> voluntarily handed it over. He seemed to respect the
> doctor's authority.

Someone else may have the voice of authority in your
loved one's life—the insurance company, a solicitor or the
Department of Transport. If this is the case, enlist their
help. Stress the importance of safety for both your relative
and other people.

If necessary, your GP can notify the Driver Vehicle
Licensing Centre. The DVLC has a division which deals

confidentially with enquiries about disabilities affecting a person's fitness to drive.

If your loved one lives alone but still has a desire to get out and about, you'll need to provide for transportation that is safe. Sharing the responsibility with family members, friends and neighbours can ease the burden. Taxi services or bus concessions may be an economical alternative in some areas. Both Alzheimer's sufferers and carers should qualify for half-price disabled travel on British Rail and London Underground. Inquire about transportation options through your local social services or through community organizations that serve the elderly. Regular routes that transport people to and from day centres, for example, might help meet your loved one's need for socialization and nutrition as well as the need to be 'on the go.'

If you hire home-care workers and feel it is safe for your loved one to ride in a car, consider employing at least one aide who is willing to drive and is appropriately licensed and insured. If you hire through an agency, check its transportation policies. Some agencies will not allow employees to transport but may forget to tell you this when you apply for help.

You may never have thought of yourself as adventurous. A spouse with Alzheimer's may change all that—particularly if getting out and going places is important to you. If you don't drive and want to learn, find out about taking lessons. Learning to drive at age fifty-five or sixty is not impossible or impractical. In fact, it may be the best gift you can give yourself both now and for the future.

Finally, *treat* your loved one. Say, 'It's time you relaxed and enjoyed the view,' as one carer successfully told her husband. You may discover that you both will actually enjoy yourselves and the scenery for the first time in months.

Remember, driving is a learned activity that quickly becomes unlearned. It's therefore a dangerous activity for someone with Alzheimer's. Driving is also a habit. Like all habits, if it's not practised, it soon fades away. It's important that it fades before any serious or tragic injuries occur.

Home Safety

Safety in and around the house is always a concern for the older person, especially the older person who lives alone. Add any degree of confusion and disorientation and the potential for disaster is multiplied.

> We no longer wanted to leave my mother alone, not for even a little while. We were always afraid she'd start a fire with her smoking. She'd light the wrong end of the cigarette sometimes and try to put it in her mouth. She'd also drop cigarettes when they were lit or stuff them in the corners of the couch to put them out. She had a plastic tablecloth on the kitchen table that was covered with cigarette burns.

> We had a pile of wood in the garage, and one day we found my father trying to light it with a blow torch. We took the torch away. Anything we thought might be dangerous we took away.
>
> One day we found Dad turning on the fire on the gas cooker. You know those inspection lights you use, the ones at the end of a long cord? Well, we'd bought one, a good one, and Dad had it. He'd cut it all up into pieces and was trying to weld it together again with the flames of the cooker.
>
> When I tried to take it away from him, he shouted at me for buying something 'cheap and inferior.' He told me it was no good.
>
> All I can say is, you have to be alert!

What is a safety hazard for one person may not be a hazard for another. An iron may present no problem to a man who has never ironed in his life. An older woman may not feel the urge to rummage through her husband's toolbox.

We don't have to totally reconstruct our houses, but we do have to know our loved one's habits. We have to be alert. Decide what are potential hazards for your relative, remembering that these may change as the disease progresses. Here are some specific situations to consider:

Prevent burns from fire, water, electricity

- Lock up electrical equipment such as hair dryers and electric shavers if there is danger that the person you care for may plug them in and drop them in the sink or bath.

- Turn down the temperature of your water heater if your loved one can no longer judge hot from cold.

- Monitor smoking by keeping matches and lighters in your possession. Many carers have found that breaking a life-long habit of smoking was unexpectedly easy for someone with Alzheimer's. Cigarettes, cigars and pipes that are out of sight may quickly fade out of mind as well.

- Remove knobs from your gas cooker or turn off the shut-off valve at night if your relative wanders and tries to cook.

- Unplug electrical appliances in the kitchen. Consider coverings for electrical outlets.

- Have a fire extinguisher in your kitchen that can be used

for all types of fires. Install smoke detectors in appropriate places and test them regularly.

- Plan escape routes from the various rooms in your house in case there is ever a need to evacuate.

Minimize cuts and bruises

- Lock up knives, power tools and other sharp objects.

- Pad the corners of sharp pieces of furniture.

- Check glassware and other dishes periodically for cracks.

Avoid accidental poisoning

- Keep medications in a safe, dry place, not in a kitchen cabinet or the bathroom medicine closet. If necessary, lock them up.

- Lock up poisonous cleaning supplies or store them in inaccessible places.

- Be aware of the signs of poisoning, which may include any of the following:

      nausea, vomiting, diarrhoea
      severe abdominal pain, cramping
      slow breathing and slow pulse
      profuse sweating or salivation
      obvious burns or stains around the mouth
      odours on the breath, such as paraffin or turpentine
      unconsciousness
      convulsions

- Keep the phone number of the ambulance next to your phone. Remember to take any empty tablet bottles or containers with you to show what has been swallowed, if you do need to go to hospital.

Decrease the danger of falls

Falls become more problematic as Alzheimer's disease progresses and areas of the brain controlling muscles and co-ordination are affected.

The following tips can help accident-proof your home against falls.

- Avoid high-gloss waxing of vinyl or wood floors.

- Eliminate loose rugs or else anchor them firmly, especially in the bathroom.

- Make sure all electrical and phone cords are outside traffic areas.

- Get rid of chairs that tip over easily. Solid and familiar furniture, strategically placed, can be an ambulation aid.

- Clear away clutter, especially on stairs.

- Remove raised doorway thresholds and replace them with flat, flush stripping.

- Put locks at the top or bottom of cellar and exit doors. Lock windows if necessary or disguise them with curtains. Alarms can also be installed on windows and doors.

- Store frequently used items on easily reached shelves.

- Light up nocturnal trips from bedroom to toilet with a 25-watt soft-light bulb, or consider night-lights in various rooms.

- Install safety bars in areas around toilet, bath and shower. Use suction mats or non-slip bath strips in bath and shower.

- Periodically check the soles and heels of shoes and slippers for wear. Thin, worn soles can be slippery.

- Avoid long hems and trailing sleeves in your relative's nightwear.

- Falls most frequently occur on the top or bottom stair step. Paint both steps in contrasting colours or use bright paint strips.

- Make certain stair railings are solid and secure.

- Block the bottom and top of the stairwell with a sturdy gate, if needed.

- Outside, make sure your entryway is well lit, any dangerous areas are well secured and pavements are in good repair.

- If your loved one needs help walking, consider purchasing a stick or Zimmer walking frame. Another possibility is a walking belt. (This can also be used to help get a person in and out of a chair or bed with minimal effort on the part of the carer.) Ask the physiotherapist or district nurse for a demonstration.

Finally, if the person you care for should fall, don't panic. Be especially careful if you attempt to break the fall. Take time to assess the situation. It may be an emergency, but chances are it is not life-threatening.

If for any reason you suspect a fracture or head injury, do not attempt to move your loved one. Simply make him or her as comfortable as possible. Use a blanket to prevent chilling, and use a rolled up blanket or pillow to support an injured limb. Then call the ambulance for help. Don't ask friends or neighbours to help you move your relative to a more comfortable position; this could cause further damage to a fractured limb.

Signs of a fracture include:

> pain or tenderness in the injured area that increases
>   with pressure or movement
> deformity—for example, a fractured hip may
>   cause one leg to appear shorter and to rotate outward
> swelling (not always immediate)
> discolouration or bruising
> exposed bone ends that have broken through the skin
> possible shock (cold, pale, clammy skin; rapid pulse;
>   shallow breathing).

If you don't suspect a fracture but are not sure you can help your loved one on your own, get help. Call a neighbour or the police.

Falling can be a symptom of other problems such as medication side-effects, poor vision, small strokes, low blood pressure,and so on. A physical examination may be in order if you notice any obvious and sudden changes in your loved one's ability to navigate around the house.

Educate Yourself and Be Prepared

Investing in a good first-aid manual can help you feel more confident if an emergency should arise. You might also want to purchase a first-aid kit or have the following supplies on hand:

> adhesive plasters
> large and small sterile gauze dressings
> crêpe bandages
> surgical adhesive tape
> scissors and safety pins
> a triangular bandage
> an eye bath
> ice packs you can keep in the freezer

Home safety for the person with Alzheimer's is much the same as home safety for anyone else: a little common sense, a little foresight into possible hazards, and a little knowledge of what to do and when to do it.

When the Emergency Is You

'In the event of an emergency,' I told one of the agency helpers I'd hired, 'I can be reached at my work phone number.'

'Fine,' she said. 'But what if the emergency is you? What if you get hit by a bus or your car lands in a ditch? What do I do with your mother?'

I had never really thought about it.

As carers for people with Alzheimer's, we hope and pray we won't ever wind up as a medical or surgical emergency, but that possibility is always present. Contrary to what most of us would like to believe, we're not immune from our own disasters or even deaths.

There's a good motto for carers who find themselves thinking about their own mortality: be prepared.

Emergency numbers

If aides care for your loved one in your home while you are away, the substitute carers should know how to reach you. Provide them with a list of emergency phone numbers that might include:

> relative(s), friend(s), neighbour(s)
> your GP; your relative's GP
> the hospital accident and emergency department
> ambulance
> police
> fire department.

Substitute carers need to know who will be responsible for your loved one should you suddenly become incapacitated. Who, specifically, should they call?

They should also have the social services number in case no one on their list can be contacted and emergency caring arrangements need to be made.

Keep a list of emergency numbers at home even if you don't hire help. It will be available in times of need.

If your loved one stays at a day centre, you will need to tell the staff where you can be reached and provide information about what to do if something should happen to you.

Emergency-care notebooks

Some carers (myself included) keep a notebook of all the vital information someone else would need in order to assume caring responsibilities in case of an emergency.

Setting aside a few hours to organize such a notebook will be well worth the effort and can contribute to your peace of mind. A notebook may prove an invaluable resource if a substitute carer comes into your home to look after your relative. It can also benefit carers in a residential home or nursing-home setting. Your notebook might include some of the following information.

Daily routine. If the person you care for has a daily routine, it's wise to include this in as much detail as possible. For example, '7:00—Usually wakes up. 7:15—Help out of bed to bedside commode. 7:30—Give sponge bath and dress.' What can your loved one do independently? What do you you have to help with?

Nutritional needs. What are your relative's eating habits and problems? Are there favourite foods? Dislikes? Allergies? Is there a favourite area to eat in? Any special dishes or cutlery? Can your relative feed himself or herself? Does he or she snack during the day?

Sleep patterns. What is the normal bedtime routine? Are naps common? If night-time wandering is a problem, what do you do to manage this behaviour?

Toileting concerns. If there's a special toileting routine to prevent or control incontinence, include details for both bladder and bowel habits.

Medications. What medications are taken? Include the name of each drug, dosage and time to be taken. Does the person you care for swallow pills without difficulty, or do pills have to be crushed and given in food or drink?

Special behaviour problems. If there are any specific problems such as wandering or 'sundowning', include these. (See chapter six for additional examples.)

Social history. Jot down anything that will make communication with your relative easier—the name he or she likes to be called, information about likes, dislikes, interests, occupation. Help the substitute carer know your loved one as a person to relate to, not a problem to solve.

Watching Over Your Loved One

It is impossible to prepare for every calamity that might occur in our lives as carers. But several additional safety measures can provide important safeguards against the unknown.

For example, if your own health is frail, consider installing an emergency-response unit at home that can be attached to your telephone. Commonly known as 'life-lines,' these units can be activated at the press of a button (usually carried or worn). Some local councils provide them free for elderly and infirm people.

Identification jewellery can be especially vital for your loved one, should the two of you be involved in an accident or should you suddenly become ill.

If you suddenly need to go to the hospital and there is no time to make emergency arrangements, insist that your loved one go with you. Have the hospital social worker notified en route or upon arrival, so special arrangements can be made for his or her care. Carry emergency numbers with you in a wallet or purse.

It is sometimes wise planning to arrange for someone to have power of attorney over you as well as over your loved one, in case you become incapacitated. Talk with your solicitor or Citizens' Advice Bureau about this. You may also wish to appoint someone else as an authorized agent to collect pensions and benefits from the Post Office, if you find it difficult to get out.

It's never pleasant to think of our own ill health, but

denial of the possibility is guaranteed to bring future grief should we suddenly become dependent.

Plan ahead. Be prepared.

Part Three

CARING FOR YOURSELF

The deepest lessons come out of the deepest waters and the hottest fires.

ELISABETH ELLIOT, *A PATH THROUGH SUFFERING*

CHAPTER TEN

People Who Help

I have always thought of myself as an active person. My solo lifestyle has meant a full-time job plus numerous activities outside the home. Moving back home to care for two older parents with health problems (my father was diagnosed with cancer) threatened to change all that. I found myself calling out for help.

When it came to affording expensive private care, my parents and I were not very wealthy. Also, many services available in more metropolitan areas were simply not available in our predominantly rural area. I realized that creative and cost-effective measures were in order if I wanted to maintain my own emotional and physical health. Caring can take its toll on both.

A verse in the New Testament book of Galatians begins, 'Carry each other's burdens.' There are many burdens we can help each other carry. As carers, we need other people to help us. We need to learn to lean.

Leaning on others is not a sign of weakness. Admitting we need other people to help us occasionally can be a sign of strength—as well as a great relief. Allowing others to help us strengthens us for our caring responsibilities.

Help can come in many forms and from a surprising

number of places. This section looks at a variety of support systems available to the carer and offers some suggestions for using them. Caring is hard, but it doesn't have to be an unbearable burden. There are many ways to lighten the load.

Support Groups

My mother wandered, never slept at night, and repeated the same words and phrases dozens of times a day. But it was my father who needed help most. Mother was well taken care of, but my dad suffered from frayed emotions, fatigue and a flagging spirit.

Dad needed a support group. And when I moved back home to help him care for my mother, I found that I needed one too.

Shortly after I returned home, a letter in our newspaper gave the phone number for a local Alzheimer's support group. I called the number and talked with one of the support-group members for over an hour. She invited me to a meeting and encouraged me to take Mum to a doctor who was willing to do a complete physical examination, including a variety of blood tests and a CAT scan. She said we'd both be better able to cope if we knew what we were dealing with and could share our concerns with others.

She was right.

Local organized support or self-help groups are scattered all over the country wherever family members provide care. They meet in homes, hospitals, nursing homes, churches. They come in all shapes and sizes, adapting themselves to the various needs represented by group members. Some are formal, with well-structured programmes. Others are informal discussions. Some are a combination of the two.

Regardless of their structure, support groups are made up of other people who can prop you up when you are weary.

When I called the local support group I discovered that Dad and I weren't alone. There were many other people in the county, some even in our own neighbourhood, who really understood our situation. They were *in* our situation.

> Sometimes you feel like you're the only person in the world with a family situation like yours. And then you go to a support-group meeting and you realize there are other people very much like you.

———————

> Sometimes I get very lonely. I have friends, but they're not the same as the friends I've made through the support group. I find I need both.

Support groups can contribute to our own emotional and spiritual well-being:

> After a while you begin to wonder if you're seeing things in the proper perspective. You feel like you're dealing with something all by yourself. But when you're able to talk with other people and listen to their experiences, you realize you're still okay yourself. You're not going off the deep end.

———————

> The support group was a place where I could share my real feelings. Even the negative ones—my guilt and my pain. No one ever said, 'You shouldn't feel that way.' No one ever said it because they all knew exactly what I was feeling. And why.

———————

Support groups can offer us more than just a listening ear. Often their help comes in very practical, material ways:

The generosity of the support group overwhelmed me. They raised the money for our travel and the overnight stay in a hotel when I had to take my husband to a research centre to be involved in an experimental drug trial.

We laugh a lot in our support group. Not at our loved ones, but at some of the things they do. Many things are funny, though usually not at the time. Then we're usually angry and frustrated. But after it's all over we need to be able to share. And to laugh. You can't do that with everyone. Some people would get offended and would think we have some sick sense of humour. But most of us realize laughter is therapy.

Support groups can even help with difficult decisions, such as whether to institutionalize or request a post-mortem:

The support group guided me to a special psychiatric hospital where my husband is now. One support-group member, who knew I couldn't face the fact that my husband needed institutionalization, said to me, 'Have you considered the psychiatric hospital? My wife has been there for ten years and she has received excellent care. Don't let preconceptions about 'mental institutions' prevent you from looking into it.'

I visited that hospital. I never would have done that without encouragement. It's a great place.

Through the support group I first heard about the need for post-mortems and how to make arrangements.

The group helped me sort through my feelings and make a decision.

Support groups are not just for carers whose loved ones are still living. Many groups include surviving spouses and relatives. Their reasons for continued involvement are varied.

My wife died four years ago and I still go to the support group. I feel that, having gone through all this, maybe I can help someone else. I think that's the way we all feel who have lost spouses or parents. Our trials are over, but maybe we can help someone whose trials aren't.

———————————

The support group fulfills a need in me to help other people. I hope that the little I can share can help relieve the problems of others.

Support groups aren't just for people who care for loved ones at home. Many carers whose loved ones are in nursing homes or hospitals continue to attend meetings.

There are a lot of people who come to our support group who have relatives in nursing homes. Sometimes visiting loved ones in a nursing home is harder than if they were home with you. It's a different kind of hard. We still need support.

———————————

The group I belong to actually meets in the nursing home where my mother is staying. It's great. The social worker leads it and we have the opportunity to ask questions. They bring in different speakers and we learn a lot. It's a nice group of people.

Support groups aren't something you should feel obligated to join. There may be a wrong time or a right time to take part:

> My first experience at a local group meeting was traumatic. I didn't want to hear about what might happen to my husband. He wasn't that bad yet, and I couldn't face the thought that he might be tied to a chair all day, playing with his shoelaces. He was still driving at the time and I just didn't want to hear how bad it was going to be. I went to the group once and then came back, a year later. Then I was ready to hear.

> I'm a very private person. I just can't share my feelings in a group. I went once and felt uncomfortable. But I do keep in touch with several of the support-group members. That helps a lot.

Groups can be helpful even if you don't think you'd be comfortable voicing your concerns in front of others, or if you simply can't get out because of caring responsibilities.

> I wasn't able to get out to the support group for two years; I didn't have anyone to care for my wife. So the group came individually and visited me. I will always be grateful.

As these carers have mentioned, most support groups have members who are willing to talk on the telephone, send information or channel you to appropriate resources and literature. They can also offer suggestions on management issues and other carer concerns, like finances and nursing-home placement. And sometimes group members do make home visits to encourage carers who cannot come to meetings.

To find out about support groups in your area, contact the Alzheimer's Disease Society or a local Age Concern office. They can help you start a support group if there are none in your area.

Support groups aren't just for adults. They can also include teenagers. If there are a number of carers with teenagers, consider establishing a separate group for the young people. If guidance is needed it might be available through a group member or someone else in the community such as a minister or a psychologist, psychotherapist or counsellor. You could also ask for help from Youth Access (see Appendix D for the address). Bringing teenagers and parents together for an informal picnic or shared supper might be a good place to start.

Last, support groups can help you feel more in control of what seems to be an uncontrollable situation. They can help you get actively engaged in the battle against Alzheimer's in a variety of ways:

> Our local group does a lot in the community. We sponsor workshops, supply speakers for churches and service clubs, distribute literature at health fairs and even our county fair. We help educate the community and increase awareness.

> Through the support group I learned how to be more involved politically, how I could take my experience of pain and make a small difference in the world. I've written letters to politicians about the financial needs of Alzheimer's families. Then I went to some meetings of the community health council. I'm now glad I first plucked up the courage to speak publicly about it.

The motto of the Alzheimer's Association in America is 'Someone to stand by you.' The motto for local support groups here could well be 'Someone to walk with you.' That is what Alzheimer's support groups have to offer.

Friends and Relations

Some carers report that their circle of friends has become more restricted as a result of their loved ones' illness. Others have discovered many new friendships. One thing is certain for all: if it weren't for friends to confide in, caring would be a very lonely business.

> I have a wonderful friend I can go to at any time. It started three years ago when she fell and broke her hip. After she came home from the hospital, I went every day and helped her put on her shoes and stockings. Sometimes I'd go early in the morning before my husband got out of bed. Other times I'd take him with me. I'd wash her feet, maybe cut her toenails, and we'd talk. She told me once, 'I want to pay you for helping me.' And I said to her, 'Are you crazy? Don't you know how much a good psychiatrist costs? I should be paying you!' She is wonderful. She simply listens.

Neighbours and relatives can also be helpful when we need a short break in the day's care.

> I had a neighbour who was very good to us. I'd take my wife over once a week and she'd just sit and watch TV. She was no trouble at all, the neighbour said. No trouble at all.

───────────────

> Our neighbour always had an open door, which was

good because my mother wandered through it a lot!
The neighbour just sat her down, got her a cup of
coffee and called us to say my mother was there and all
right.

My daughter-in-law's a hairdresser. Every Saturday
she does my wife's hair at her house, which is not the
easiest thing to do because my wife gets up about five
or six times and wanders around. That's my break
time. It's the only chance I get during the week to mow
the lawn or to talk on the phone without getting inter-
rupted.

Sometimes friends and neighbours might avoid us. Often
this happens because of their own emotional response to
Alzheimer's disease, not because of an uncaring attitude or
rudeness.

Visits with a person with Alzheimer's may remind our
friends and neighbours of their own advancing age and
mortality, two things many people would like to forget.
Reasons for what carers perceive to be fair-weather friends
or neglectful neighbours vary:

I really wanted to visit, but I didn't do it very much. I
know my best friend's wife thought it was a lack of
caring on my part. It wasn't. I was just plain scared.
Now that he's dead I feel guilty. What can I say?

The same may be true of relatives who you may feel have
abandoned your sinking ship and are shirking their responsibility. Carers often express feelings of anger, resentment
and frustration because of perceived abandonment. However, relatives may simply be unable to face their own fears
and their loved one's failing health and frailty.

157

You should have seen my wife's brother. He was hotter than blazes when he found out she was in a nursing home. When he finally went up and saw her, she didn't know him. He said to me, 'I didn't know she was this bad.' I said, 'I've been trying to tell you for three years, but you wouldn't believe me.' Later he told me he didn't *want* to believe it.

––––––––––––

It bothers me that my oldest child hasn't been to see his grandmother in over three years. But he can't seem to take it. He gets emotional when he's there and he starts to cry. And he's thirty-eight years old. On one hand, I think he should make himself go. But then, I suppose, she doesn't know him anyway. Maybe it doesn't matter.

––––––––––––

In our case it's been much harder for the two oldest siblings to visit. They can't face it. In a dire emergency they might be of help, but not now, not on a steady basis. They're dealing with their own concerns about their future and also their own hurt and pain in facing the current situation. I know it's very painful. I hurt too. It's especially hard on my father and mother.

––––––––––––

My brother lives in another state and, when he calls, he never talks about Dad. He keeps it inside.

One day he did visit, and he went with us to the nursing home. He didn't want to go but I said to him, 'You've been away for several years and you have no idea what's going on. I think it would be a good idea if you went out to see Dad. In fact, maybe you think it's a lot more gruesome than it actually is.'

So my brother went with us and we sat and talked to Dad, or, rather, my mother and I sat and talked to Dad. I don't think my brother could understand how we could be so cool about it. We talked and laughed and fed Dad lunch while the kids were in the background, banging on the piano. My brother just sat and watched us and didn't say a word. At one point I said, 'Are you glad you came?' and he said, 'Yes,' and that was the end of that.

It's sad because I think my brother has been dying inside all these years. His best friend says he won't talk about it to him either. Maybe he's handling it. I hope so.

We'd all like to think that a chronic illness like Alzheimer's would bring families and friends closer together, not pull them apart. It can do both, depending to some extent on our attitudes as carers and our willingness to understand and help our other loved ones. We may, at times, have to be gentle and forgiving in the midst of our own emotional upheavals. Life is too short and relationships are too valuable to carry grudges.

Yet sometimes the problem isn't difficulty dealing with emotions at all. Not everyone is comfortable being a carer or being around people who are physically or mentally impaired. Families and friends may not know what they can do. They may feel awkward. Or they may want to help but fear they'll be invading our privacy. Sometimes they need us to give them permission to help us. We can do this by asking them for assistance or advice.

There are many ways friends and relations can offer support to their loved one and to the primary carer. One carer told me how her whole family gets involved in her mother's care, even though they are separated by distance. Geography doesn't seem to be a barrier for this family. Though distance precludes day-to-day care, they make periodic visits and work together as a team.

The son is the problem solver. He uses his expertise to help with financial and legal problems. One sister is the 'organizer'. She helped get her parents Meals-on-Wheels and a place at the day centre, and she organized information about an experimental-drug programme her mother became involved with.

Another is the practical manager. She takes her mother shopping when she visits, alters clothing and takes home special laundry, helping in practical ways.

A third sister is the sounding board, the listener. She visits for a month at a time, offering encouragement and emotional support.

Sometimes this support springs up naturally and spontaneously. In other situations, it's good to have a family planning conference early in the disease process. This will help identify and co-ordinate the skills family members can contribute as the disease progresses and their loved one's needs increase.

- Contributing to loved ones' financial needs is one way some relatives can share in the caring burden. Caring is expensive. Even if most of the expense is covered by the National Health or social services there are always items of extra expense, for example, some incontinence products, special foods, wheelchair repair, not to mention respite care.

- Family members living in other parts of the country often attend support groups themselves. This gives them a more realistic picture of what the primary carer is coping with and what their loved one is suffering. In addition, they can learn more about Alzheimer's disease by attending conferences and exchanging audio tapes. Information they acquire can be shared across the miles.

- Never underestimate the value of letters and phone calls. For the primary carer the feeling of aloneness doesn't lessen as the years go by—no matter how involved one may be in the community or in a support group. Tangible notes of support and encouragement help maintain and strengthen family ties.

Caring really is a family affair. It is a time for sharing and bearing each other's burdens in practical, tangible ways.

Little Ones

My five-year-old grandson loves his grandmother. When my daughter takes him to the nursing home to visit, he'll climb up on my wife's lap and kiss her. Then she'll smile, just like old times. He's the only one who can make her smile like that. He can be out in the hall and my wife will recognize his voice. She'll even shout to the nurses, 'That's my boy. Let him come!' My wife always calms down when he comes.

I told my grandson that I wished we could have his grandmother back home again with us. You know what he said to me? He said, 'That's all right, Grandpa. Grandma's poorly. But that doesn't stop me from loving her.'

Newborns. Infants. Toddlers. School-age children. Teenagers. If you have any children in your family or can borrow some from your friends, they can be a source of joy for both you and your loved one. Relating to your loved one can likewise be a joy for them.

Occasionally children will be frightened by their grandmother's or grandfather's bizarre behaviour, but most of the time they'll take it in stride and accept it.

Mum and her four-year-old grandson get along just fine. To a four-year-old, everything is new in the world and everything is as it should be. Therefore, if Grandma is confused and forgetful, that's okay. It must be normal. We'll accept that behaviour. And so he does.

When I hired some carers for my mother several years ago, one of the workers had two children, ages seven and nine. She brought them to work in the summer, and they always came along after school during the school year. Mum called them 'cute little fellers' (a phrase she also uses when referring to the squirrels on our patio and even some of my older friends). But they didn't seem to mind. She also patted them on the head a lot and gave them hugs. They accepted her terms of endearment and responded in kind. To them, she was 'Gramma.'

Once I got home from work and discovered Mum and the two children hard at work on a special project that the children themselves had instituted. They'd brought over their colouring books and had also bought one for my mum. The three of them were having a great time colouring at the kitchen table. My mother the artist was once again at work.

As the months went by, my mother lost her ability to hold on to crayons. While her colouring lasted, it was a joy to watch her interact with the children for even short periods of time and to see the children care about her, accepting some of Mum's other behaviour as a normal part of life for a 'grandmother' with Alzheimer's.

A week before my father died, one of the children wrote my mother a letter. It seems a fitting reminder of the importance of children in the lives of our relatives—a reminder of what love is all about:

Dear Pearl

Hi How are you today. I love you a lot. You are my best Friend. You are more Than a Friend. you are Like a Grama to me and all way be a Grama to me Because I Love you so much. you will all ways Be in my Heart. you are so Loveable & soft and so warm. and you allways will be in my Heart and in my Dreams. an so Does God Love you Like I Do. He will allways watch over you pearl because I love you. and I love God to.

From Tanya L. Rood to pearl

CHAPTER ELEVEN

Get Me Out of Here!

Elaine remembered when she loved her job. When it had been, in fact, her respite. But lately the tensions at work were unbearable. There was always the constant backbiting and bickering. And there were the stupid, hateful things the other women said about their husbands. If they only knew, Elaine thought bitterly. If they only knew. They should be grateful they have husbands.

They should come home with me, she thought. See what it's like to live with a husband who doesn't even know your name. They'd begin to appreciate what they've got in a hurry. I wonder if anyone would take me up on the offer if I did invite them home.

Home. Thinking of home, Elaine wondered how the new home-care helper was getting on. The previous one lasted only a week. She turned in her resignation to the agency the day Stephen locked her out of the house. He had somehow managed to unlock the kitchen door in the morning and run out into the back garden. When the helper ran after him, Stephen ran around the house and back into the kitchen, slamming and locking the door.

The woman spent two hours pleading with Stephen to let her in. But Stephen just stood there, smiled, and waved at her. When the helper saw him turn the gas on under an empty frying pan, she had the presence of mind to run to the neighbour's house and call the police. And then she rang her agency.

Despite the problems, Elaine didn't know what she'd have done without the home-care agency. The helpers had been so good to Stephen. One of them even joked about losing ten pounds the first week she cared for him. It made Elaine feel guilty until the carer reassured her it was the best thing to happen to her figure in years.

But people in their forties weren't supposed to *need* minders. They weren't supposed to get Alzheimer's disease. Cancer maybe, or diabetes or a heart attack. Terrible things, too, but all potentially treatable. Not Alzheimer's. Not this horrible disease that turned you into some kind of hyperactive child.

When had it first begun? When did she first notice the signs?

It wasn't until Stephen received the letter from the school requesting his resignation that reality finally hit her.

The absent-minded professor, the kids called Stephen at school. At first it showed in little things. He would correct their essays and forget to give them marks. Then he went through one term without giving an exam at all. The pupils never told. The school governors accidentally found out about Stephen's memory lapses when one of the governors overheard his daughter talking to a friend about the strange and wonderful chemistry teacher.

Finally the day came when, in the middle of chemistry lab, Stephen threw a beaker at a student in a fit of frustration. Fortunately, the only thing in the beaker was water. It should have been acid; Stephen had forgotten the formula.

Now Elaine could look back and see other changes. There were initially problems with words. Stephen always seemed to be searching to find the noun or the phrase to end a sentence. It started to drive Elaine crazy. Half the time she didn't know what he was talking about.

And there were personality changes. The frustration. The angry outbursts for no apparent reason.

She remembered the Saturday morning Stephen went to the shops for a pint of milk and returned six hours later. She had really laid into him, accusing him of everything under the sun. And Stephen just looked at her, then went into the bedroom, slammed and locked the door and stayed there until after dark. That happened just before they got the letter from the school governers.

Two years later, here they were. Alone in a world where nothing made sense any more.

Maybe she should have listened to her mother and had a child. But no. She and Stephen had both felt that all they wanted was each other and their careers. They were planning to take a trip around the world in three more years. No strings. No children. Each other.

Elaine opened her desk and reached for her purse. Time to go home. Home to the man she still loved beyond distraction and who didn't even know her name.

Let's see. Purse. Leftover lunch. Library book. Bible.

Bible. Yes. She really should take that home with her and read it, Elaine thought. Especially those verses in the book of Isaiah. Once they were all that kept her sane, kept her going. But lately she'd got out of the habit of reading. Still, Elaine carted the Bible to the office each day, thinking that maybe *this* lunch hour she would find some time. She certainly never found time at home.

Where was that passage? Ah, yes. Isaiah 54. 'Your creator will be like a husband to you . . . " . . .I will show you my love for ever." So says the Lord who saves you.'

The Lord, her husband.

Not Stephen. Not any more. At least not in the sense that he could meet her needs for friendship or companionship. Not Stephen, her husband, but the Lord, her maker.

As Elaine slipped the Bible into her handbag, she fervently prayed that when she walked through her kitchen door in forty-five minutes, she would remember what she had read—and have hope for her own life.

Feeling the Pressure

You may think, as a number of carers have told me, that no one can care for your loved one as well as you can. This may be true. But if you are a parent you probably said the same thing when you first left your child with a baby sitter or sent your first child off to nursery school. Much to your amazement, you both survived. You will survive this time too.

> Dad was very aggressive. He mellowed somewhat as he got older, but his temper got worse as the Alzheimer's disease came on. It was very hard on my mother. She was the type of person who would take everything and wouldn't fight back. But there were times when she would go into her room, shut the door, cry, and scream and scream—just to get rid of the tension. I don't know why she didn't have a nervous breakdown. Ten years, and no respite.

As Alzheimer's disease progresses, most carers will need some short-term relief as well as extended periods of respite. Friends or family members may be willing to fill in for long weekends. An extended getaway, however, requires more formal arrangements. A number of options are available to carers depending on where you live, your financial situation and your needs.

Using all the available community services and care providers make can it possible for us to keep our loved one at home for as long as it is safe and desirable. They are not designed to totally take away our caring responsibilities but to give us the short-term help we need to rest, regroup and recoup our personal strength and resources. We are then better equipped to manage at home when we return.

Home Care

Formal in-home services delivered through city, regional and community agencies include various types of nursing services, home-care helpers, 'sitters', respite workers and home helps/housekeepers. Mealtime help may be provided through Meals-on-Wheels or other nutrition programmes that provide meals to people with disabilities.

Carers frequently cite the value of regularly scheduled home-care workers:

> Helpers from a local home-care agency came in twice a week to give my husband a bath, shave him and give him his breakfast. After breakfast, they'd take him for a walk. It was so good to have a couple of hours to myself.

> _____

> I'm semi-retired and have a part-time teaching job two afternoons a week. I asked some volunteers from the Crossroads Care to come in when I finally realized I had to have someone with her when I was at work. My major support came from these volunteers.

> _____

> Home care was wonderful. It was my salvation. The girl who came was great. And I worked outside the home every day, five days a week.
> My work was really my respite. I couldn't have stood being home all day long.

If you're looking for in-home services, the following tips may apply:

Talk with other carers who have hired helpers. What services have they used? Were the services reliable and dependable?

Ring your department of social services who can tell you what is available in your area. It is also well worth contacting your local Alzheimer's group, Age Concern representative, Women's Royal Voluntary Service or other community organization and explaining your needs. Even if the people that you contact are unable to provide services directly, they should be able to refer you to agencies that can.

Statutory health care can vary according to area, but may include a community psychiatric nurse (CPN) who can offer invaluable heap and advice. A district nurse should be able to assist with bathing, dressing and other practical concerns. Sometimes a health visitor may fill this role. Twilight Nursing Services are sometimes available to help in putting a confused elderly person to bed.

Crossroads Care is a voluntary agency that provides an attendant care service to more than 12,000 British families. It is designed to supplement the existing provision for care by the social services. Enquire whether a Crossroads scheme operates in your area.

If you need home-care help following the hospital discharge of your loved one, contact the hospital's social worker as soon as possible. This person can help you make post-hospital arrangements and is also a good agency-referral source.

If you can afford it, there are a number of advantages to hiring through an established, reputable agency. These may include training and supervision of home-care workers, development of a specific plan of care, provision of substitute workers if the scheduled worker is ill, and provision of various levels of service ranging from cooking, cleaning and shopping to direct personal caring.

Turn the above advantages into questions for the agency when you ask about information and services.

It helps if written information is available about the agency's services, certification, fees and funding sources.

Most sufferers from dementia are eligible for Attendance Allowance, and some for Mobility Allowance and Invalid Care Allowance. Details of these benefits are in the Disability Rights Handbook (obtainable from the Disability Alliance and from the Alzheimer's Disease Society). Benefits change, and a Welfare Rights Adviser, who can be contacted through the local Citizens' Advice Bureau, will be able to help you in these matters.

The Alzheimer's Disease Society has also established a Caring Fund from which small grants are made to those in need, as a supplement to state benefits.

Many home-care expenses are tax deductible for spouses and children who are primary carers. Be sure to save all medically related receipts and keep accurate records of expenses.

If agency help is not available or affordable, as is often the case, you can also hire on an individual basis. Many men and women with kind hearts and good skills are looking for home-care jobs. These people may have been trained through on-the-job experience with home-care agencies, or in hospitals or nursing homes.

Newspapers may have adverts from home-care workers seeking independent employment. These workers may be trained or certified aides, though training itself is not necessarily an indication of how reliable or how honest an aide will be. Avoid hiring over the phone. It's best to have applicants come to your home for a personal interview. Are they able to physically manage your loved one? Find out about any health problems. Will they need to do heavy lifting? Can they? Discuss fees (they will usually set an hourly rate) based on what they want, what you can afford and what you believe is the going rate in your area.

To minimize risks, ask prospective employees for several references, preferably previous employers. Call them. A good employee will not mind this or feel that it's an intrusion.

Communicate with other carers who may have hired help in the past. A 'carer grapevine' can let you know who's reliable and who's not.

College and hospital nursing programmes may be a useful source of home-care help. Students are often looking for part-time employment. Sometimes they are also looking for a place to live, perhaps while they take a break from their studies. For two years I had a student live with us. In exchange for room, board and a negotiated salary, she cared for my mother and enabled me to hold down a full-time job. She had weekends and evenings off but was always willing to help me out when I needed some extra time for myself.

Age Concern has published a factsheet called *Finding Help at Home* which is worth obtaining. Another useful free factsheet, *Help at Home*, may be obtained from Counsel and Care for the Elderly. The addresses may be found at the end of this book (see Appendix D). Please enclose a large stamped addressed envelope when writing.

Adult Day Centres

'If only there had been a place where I could have left my mother for the day. I simply needed a day off now and then,' said one carer. There *are* such places. Adult day-care programmes provide socialization, a nutritious meal, and a structured and supervised environment with a wide range of activities.

Availability, criteria for eligibility and the cost of day-care services vary widely from state to area to area, but they are usually a very economical—perhaps the *most* economical—form of help for the carer.

Most adult day centres are run by the local authorities or voluntary groups; others may be affiliated with and located in geriatric hospitals or nursing homes. Some centres care for all older people with physical and intellectual impairment. Others are only for those with physical disabilities or people with dementia. Payment may be means-tested.

One job I held several years ago necessitated a two-hour drive once a month for management meetings. The meeting was in a fairly large city. I inquired about day-care options and found a centre, which catered exclusively to Alzheimer's sufferers, only a mile from our meeting place. So Mum went with me on the monthly trips. She loved the run and seemed to thrive in the centre's environment.

I loved it too: eight hours later I was only a few pounds poorer. Home care would have cost me four to five times as much for the twelve hours away from home.

If you do any travelling, think about this option and ring in advance to learn about available services.

Residential care homes are another option. These are run by local authorities or voluntary groups or, increasingly, are privately run. Those run by local authorities may be called 'Part III' homes. They provide live-in, twenty-four-hour help for the frail elderly. Some exclusively take in people with Alzheimer's. Some are willing to care for people only during the day, on an occasional overnight, or for several weeks or a month of respite for needy carers. I use this option about twice a month at an affordable cost. Your social-service department will have an official listing, though you may need more information than this offers. Once again, ask around.

Another option I discovered was the 'sitter/companion.'

Many child minders don't mind another mouth to feed at lunch and, if an Alzheimer's sufferer is manageable and doesn't wander, would see him or her as a welcome addition to their home.

I use this service once a week. I drop Mum off in the morning, go to work at the nursing home and return around nine at night, taking some time for myself. I pay the regular rate. Mum seems to enjoy her times with the children, and they like to be with her. My refrigerator is covered with 'pictures for Pearle' that one little girl keeps giving us. Ask around. Check references if you need to.

Other Alternatives

You may also want to consider some of these alternative options for the care of your loved one:

Some hospitals, nursing homes and residential care homes provide respite care for carers on a short-term basis. If this service is not available in your area, your support group might consider it worth lobbying for. It can be a wonderful relief for a carer who is ill or needs a real holiday.

The Holiday Care Service is a registered charity providing free information and advice on holidays for people with special needs. Contact them direct for their booklet *Care for Carers* and a range of other useful information for carers. The address is at the back of this book.

An exchange programme with other carers in your support group may be possible. It may not be any more difficult or time consuming to care for two or even three people with Alzheimer's than to care for one. In fact, there may be *less* care involved.

At the various day centres and residential homes I've either used or visited, I've seen that people with Alzheimer's have a language all their own; they often communicate very well with each other, especially in the later stages of the disease. In fact, they may find it a relief to care for each other and talk to each other, and the carer's burden is lessened.

Keep Searching

Some carers have tried a number of the foregoing options and have had negative experiences. This is to be expected. We know that caring for someone with Alzheimer's is not easy. Not everyone can do it. Even some trained nurses may never have encountered dementia.

We needn't let one or even two or three rough experiences sour us to all substitute carers. Sooner or later we'll end up with a good match and probably wonder how we ever managed without the support of that particular home-care agency, volunteer sitter or day-care programme.

That's as it should be as we shift the caring responsibility on to someone else's shoulders for a while and take a needed break.

The Ultimate Resource

I heard a story once about a nurse who was caring for children. One little boy, confined to an oxygen tent, was not only having difficulty breathing, he was terrified by the whole experience of confinement and separation.

The nurse had a solution. She opened the tent flaps and crawled in beside the screaming toddler. Sensing her presence, the comfort of another human being, the child promptly fell asleep.

As carers, we may feel a lot like that screaming little boy. We may not have difficulty breathing, but we do have difficulty coping with the day-to-day responsibilities that threaten to overwhelm us. We feel claustrophobic, confined and terrified. We desperately long for someone to 'climb into our tents with us' and give us comfort or, better yet, set us free.

Sometimes we can escape from our emotionally charged tents for a few hours. We may get out of the house, shop, golf, dine with friends or attend a support-group meeting.

But unfortunately not all of us can get out. Even if we do, we still need support and understanding when the door closes behind us back home—where we're alone with our loved ones.

Our freedom is illusory. But there is a resource, one we might think of as our ultimate support system. I believe that our ultimate resource is God.

> I don't think anything in life would make sense without faith. I think of my father. You live your life, you're alert, you give to society, and then all of a sudden your body and mind start giving way.
>
> My father's illness wouldn't make sense without God. Without God there would be no justice.
> If I hadn't had a relationship with Jesus—a *personal* relationship—I couldn't have gone on.

We may need to be reminded at times that God truly does love us and our loved ones. He cares about our confusion and the emotional pain we have as carers. He wants to carry us through it.

CHAPTER TWELVE
Our Tangled Emotions

I remember sitting in the kitchen with my two-year-old, feeling miserable, when a song about a woman who had died started playing on the radio. I started sobbing.

My emotions were all bottled up inside. That song triggered them. I went outside, sat on the steps for half an hour and cried and cried. I couldn't stop. There was all this pent-up emotion.

I knew it was because of my mother.

Our emotional responses to Alzheimer's are often as mixed up and tangled as the minds of those we care for. Sometimes we need help to sort through them and straighten them out.

Fear, anxiety, guilt, anger and depression are the primary emotions carers experience. But the full picture needn't look so bleak. What we may perceive as negative emotions are a natural if uncomfortable response to what is really our loss of a loved one. The one we love may still be alive and present, but not as the person we knew. What we are doing, in fact, is grieving. And grief is healthy and normal.

Granger Westberg, in his popular book *Good Grief*, writes about the emotions people feel when facing the loss of a loved one. He notes that there are good and bad ways to grieve, healthy and unhealthy emotions to experience. Grief is a 'road the majority of humans must travel in order to get back into the mainstream of life.' That applies to carers.

To be free from worry and anxiety in the face of uncertainty, to be at peace with those we care for without feeling resentful or resigned—these are healthy signs that we have come to terms with our conflicting emotions. They show that we are truly experiencing 'good' grief.

Fears and Anxieties

Fear and anxiety are common emotional reactions when a relative is diagnosed with Alzheimer's. They are strongest among children of Alzheimer's sufferers.

The question 'Is Alzheimer's disease hereditary?' is asked by every son and daughter. We pray the answer is no. We fear the answer is yes. Fear and anxiety may increase if we know our family history:

> I think it may be the fourth generation for my mother. Her mother died when she was sixteen. We're sure it was Alzheimer's. My mother's grandmother had the same symptoms. Judging from the family anecdotes we've been gathering, a great-uncle had symptoms too.

The fear becomes even greater if we, too, become forgetful.

> Sometimes I forget the names of people I should know, and that terrifies me. My wife sees the look that comes over my face and she says, 'Now, don't start getting upset.'

Many carers can cope by joking about the possibility of

Alzheimer's. Others use their knowledge to plan for the future.

My two sisters and I crack jokes about how we'll be the old Alzheimer's gals. We'll get a home together.

I'm not really afraid of getting Alzheimer's. If I do, I hope I have enough lucid moments in the beginning so that I'll have time to make plans and take care of everything.

I certainly don't sit around and worry. I do, occasionally, think about planning for the future.

I kid about it with my roommate sometimes. She'll say to me, 'You're acting funny again. Sign the paper.' We make a joke of it.

I did tell her that, if I ever start acting as my father did, I want to sign the paper so someone will have power of attorney over me.

Sometimes the more we know about the disease, the less we're able to cope with it. Other people can help put our fears and anxieties in perspective.

I read some information about Alzheimer's disease that said I had a good chance of getting Alzheimer's because my mother had it. Then I went to a conference where they talked about the heredity factor. I was so depressed when I came home, I spent the next four days in bed.

A friend said, 'Are you going to make your husband and your children miserable for the next twenty years just because you think you might get it? You'll ruin

your lives. And besides, you could get
hit by a bus tomorrow. A plane could fall from the sky.
You simply can't worry about getting this disease.'

Are fear and anxiety justified? Is Alzheimer's hereditary?
What are the risks to children of Alzheimer's sufferers and
to future generations?

Studies have demonstrated an increased risk of developing Alzheimer's among those who have Alzheimer's in their
family. However, the majority of cases of the disease are *not*
genetic. In those which are, the age of onset is relatively low
(between approximately thirty-five and sixty years) and is
constant within the family. Because of this, it may be
possible to trace the disease back over several generations.
Your family is unlikely to have the inherited type of Alzheimer's unless there are at least three relatives from one side of
the family who have developed the disease before the age of
sixty. Even if that is the case, you are not at high risk unless
one of your parents is a sufferer. In those few families where
the disease is a dominant genetic disorder, about half the
children of affected parents will develop Alzheimer's.
Nevertheless, if you are already over the age of onset in your
family, you are probably no longer at risk. Remember, most
cases of the disease are *not* inherited.

Researchers are constantly looking for links between Alzheimer's and similar diseases. One area of genetic exploration
is related to Down's syndrome or mongolism, a hereditary
condition accompanied by an extra chromosome that causes
profound mental retardation.

The possible genetic thread linking both Alzheimer's
disease and Down syndrome is the presence of a large
number of senile plaques and neurofibrillary tangles present
in brain tissue of both Alzheimer's and Down's syndrome
sufferers.

Autopsies on Down's syndrome sufferers over the age of

forty show evidence of the characteristic plaques and tangles of Alzheimer's disease—even if they didn't exhibit Alzheimer's when they were alive. This finding has sparked considerable interest and activity in genetic research that may one day uncover a cause and a cure for Alzheimer's.

It is possible to be referred to a genetic counsellor through your GP if you are concerned about the inherited form of Alzheimer's disease in your family. Rather than fear the genetic implications, we should welcome scientific advances and encourage the research that may help subsequent generations.

Hope for future generations may seem scant comfort to us, struggling with the reality of Alzheimer's disease. But if God provides rain for the earth and food for the animals, he can and will provide for us. He can give us the strength to be carers today and to face the future with peace.

The Guilt Trip

Psychiatrist Karl Menninger, in his book *Whatever Became of Sin?*, describes a man who stood on a busy street corner and repeated one word aloud, over and over again. The word was *guilty*. Each time the man said 'Guilty,' he'd point at a passerby. The accused people hesitated, looked away, then glanced furtively at each other—as if they actually *felt* guilty.

Carers may feel a lot like those poor pedestrians. Whatever we say, wherever we go, whatever we do, we can't escape the pointing finger. If we don't think others are pointing it at us, we point it at ourselves. It's a no-win situation.

What makes us feel guilty? Dozens of things.

We feel guilty about our attitude toward our loved one's confusion, agitation and behaviours.

I felt guilty every minute of the day. Not so much for

the way I treated my mother, but for the things I thought about her.

I didn't holler or scream, but I certainly felt like it at times. Her agitation, and especially the repetitiveness, drove me nuts.

I usually coped by walking out of the room, leaving my mother in her chair to talk to herself. I suppose you might call that neglect, but it was the only way I could handle my emotions.

———————

I was never outright mean to my wife. I didn't physically abuse her. But I acted as if she didn't exist. She'd ask me a question for the twenty-fifth time in one morning and I'd just walk away.
Ignoring her became a habit.

I felt guilty about it, a nagging, clawing kind of guilt.

Our behaviour can bother us when we finally vent our pent-up emotions and verbally or even physically lash out in a carer's version of a catastrophic reaction.

I would be so very mean to my husband. I'd say cutting, hurtful things to him. I couldn't seem to stop myself. I was so frustrated.

———————

I would get mad at my wife and feel badly later. I don't think you can help that. You're driven to extremes, then, afterward you're sorry.

One time my wife bit me so hard I turned around and bit her on the shoulder. She had so many clothes on it didn't hurt her at all. It was just a sudden reaction on my part. Then I felt guilty.

The decision to place a relative in a nursing home is often

fraught with guilt, compounded by the promises we may have made to 'never, ever do such a thing.'

I think the hardest thing for me was taking my husband to the nursing home. He was still lucid enough to realize we were taking him away from his home, and he said, 'I worked so hard all my life. Why are you doing this to me?'

You can imagine how I felt, how I still feel.

Father used to say, 'Don't ever put me in a nursing home. Take me out in the field and shoot me before you put me in one of those places.'

So we told him we'd never do it. And then, one day, we did it.

I've read that people have taken care of their loved ones at home for seventeen years. So I felt guilty for not keeping him home.

I still feel guilty whenever I visit him, especially if he's alert.

But what could I do? I'm eighty-nine years old.

Wishing a parent, spouse, sister or brother dead and out of their misery is not an uncommon source of guilt.

When my brother was still driving, I thought that maybe he'd drive off the cliff in back of our house and it would be over for him. It would end his suffering.

I never told anyone I had those thoughts.

Once my father was lost and my brother found him

wandering down by the river. When he came home, my brother said to me, 'I had the most horrible thoughts when we were searching. I hoped that Dad might have fallen in the river and that it was all over for him. I felt so guilty for thinking that way.'

Neglected responsibilities make us feel guilty—the floors to mop, the lawn to mow, the letters to answer and the bills to pay.

I know my house is a wreck and I've let things pile up. Sometimes I get overwhelmed by depression. Most of the time I just feel guilty because I think I should be able to get my act together and keep things in order: my father, my house, my life.

———————

Our neighbours must think they live next to an abandoned building. The grass is two feet high. Garden work always seems to be at the bottom of my priority list, and I feel ashamed of the way my house looks. Inside as well as outside.

Unmet family obligations and needs can create guilt for us.

My husband was a brick through it all. Sometimes I wonder why he didn't ask for a divorce. I certainly didn't meet many of his needs for a whole year after my mother moved in with us. *Any* of his needs, if you know what I mean.

———————

It was hard on the children to grow up in the same house with a grandparent who had Alzheimer's. They never complained, but I know it was hard.

We couldn't do anything together as a family, because someone had to stay home and watch Dad. I don't think I have any pictures from a family holiday. Holidays never happened. I feel bad about that.

Psychologists may tell this carer that her guilt is false, related to the unrealistic expectations we have of ourselves. This may be true. But simply *calling* it false guilt doesn't help. And sorting false guilt from real guilt, when we're overwhelmed by both, can seem impossible.

At home we tried every day to give Dad a bath or just wash him, but he'd always fight. When we took Dad to the nursing home, he had dirt in the creases of his neck. I was embarrassed.

When I visited him and looked at his neck, it was clean. I said, 'Thank God,' but I was embarrassed again!

Sometimes we need other people to help us sort through our guilt. A friend, members of our support group, counsellors and clergy can all be valuable sounding boards.

Yet when we're all talked out, supported, analyzed, and back home again, we may find that things really haven't changed. Our guilt hasn't walked away. We still respond the same way to the same situations. Guilt continues to incapacitate us emotionally and physically. It threatens to force us into self-condemnation and depression.

Guilt, even false guilt, is never benign. And, unfortunately, false guilt can be a smoke screen. It can effectively hide an underlying problem we have apart from our caring experiences. That problem is *true* guilt.

None of us are perfect in all our actions and our attitudes.

If we deal with guilt superficially by denying it or rationalizing it, we can continue to struggle alone. But I believe that if we admit to God our deep-down failings and regrets, we can experience genuine forgiveness.

The freedom that comes from being forgiven is more than simply not feeling guilty. It is the experience of new life and the promise of life to come. It is the realization that it's possible to have joy in the midst of mourning, hope in the midst of despair. It is knowing that the experience of caring does not have to devastate us. That is indeed good news.

CHAPTER THIRTEEN

Hot But Not Burned Up

Over ten years ago I was working in a nursing home in Illinois as a spiritual-care co-ordinator. I loved my job, I loved the area, and I was *in* love. The fact that he wasn't equally in love with me was something I figured would work itself out in time. I was really looking forward to my future.

Then came the phone call.

'Sharon,' said my aunt, my father's youngest sister. 'You know you've always said to let you know if there were any problems on the home front. Well, there are. With your mother. I think it's time you moved back home.' That was not news I wanted to hear.

I knew for years that my mother was having 'a bit of a memory problem.' I attributed it to her retirement, failing eyesight and my dad's sudden onset of adult diabetes, an event that seemed to throw my mother into a state of confusion and anxiety. Alzheimer's disease was the furthest thing from my mind. I couldn't even spell it.

I received a lot of advice from friends and colleagues. Even the administrator of the nursing home called me into her office. She gave me a very comforting lecture on how I needed to think about my needs, my future, my job. Perhaps you should call your father and talk to him about the possibility of nursing-home placement, she suggested. Take a

186

short leave of absence, get things squared away at home, then come back. Neat. Simple. Just what I wanted to hear.

That was not, however, what I was supposed to do. God, it seemed, had other plans for my life. He made them clear in no uncertain terms one night when I was reading the Bible.

In the book of Mark, Jesus was speaking to the religious leaders of the day. He was talking to them about their responsibility to their parents, and he called them hypocrites. They apparently gave money for temple offerings while their parents went hungry. They were, Jesus said, worshipping God in vain.

I felt convicted and doomed. I packed my bags—not eagerly, not happily—and drove home.

For the next several years I helped my father care for my mother. I either lived at home or shuffled back and forth between my parents' home and an apartment in a nearby city where I found a nursing job. Life seemed an unending merry-go-round of work, work, and more work as Mum's symptoms got worse, my father developed cancer, and I had to face the facts that I was probably back home for good, constantly caring and still very much single.

I was also very angry with God.

My primary support system had always been my church. I stopped going. The Bible had always been my point of strength. I stopped reading. Prayer had always been my source of encouragement. I stopped praying.

It was easy to justify my lack of church involvement. I had my parents as an excuse.

It was something I tried not to think about very much; I hoped no one would ask me about it. Few did. For months I continued being both angry and miserable. Then I finally came to terms with my feelings and began dealing with them constructively.

God isn't always the target of our anger. Sometimes we're

angry at Alzheimer's itself, a disease we barely understand and cannot control.

I was angry at this disease that was destroying my father's mind. I was angry because life wasn't turning out the way I'd envisioned for my parents.

———————————

I quit smoking so I wouldn't get lung cancer. I changed my diet so I wouldn't have a heart attack. And here comes this disease that I have absolutely no control over. I can't do anything to prevent it. I realize no matter how healthy my lifestyle is, I won't be able to stop it or do anything about it if I get it. And because my mother has it, I look at myself as being a sitting duck.

It angers me. I know anger isn't going to do me any good, but it makes me so mad.

Sometimes our anger at our loved ones, then at ourselves because we don't feel good about our angry outbursts. We want to change, but we struggle.

We were angry with my mother for the things she said and did. It would be so frustrating. She would ask the same questions over and over again until my father thought he'd go out of his mind. What day is it? What day is it? What month is it? What month is it? The same questions over and over.

Dad would say, 'For Pete's sake, I told you the answer to that ten times already.' Then he'd go into the bedroom and slam the door.

———————————

There's always a tendency, especially if there are other

people around, to let your best side show, though inside you know things are different. I didn't want my patience to be a mask I was putting on.

When I got those feelings of anger and impatience, I didn't like it. Daddy knew he was irritating me. He'd try to apologize for something that wasn't his fault. I got very upset with myself for being angry and impatient with him when he'd ask me the same thing for the hundredth time.

When I got that way, I'd go into the bedroom and pray. I'd say, 'Help me to be patient. Help me to remember. Help me to show Daddy the patience I'd want someone to show me.'

Primary carers may feel they are the only ones who really care about their loved ones. Anger at other members of the family who 'never call, never visit, never show any concern,' is common.

I don't understand why my wife's brother never visits. For ten years she's had Alzheimer's. For five years she's been in the nursing home. He's never visited her there once. Not once.

In hospitals and nursing homes anger is sometimes directed at health-care staff, doctors, nurses or nursing assistants.

I got furious at some of the things the nursing auxiliaries would say or do. You can't treat people like cattle, but that's the way they behaved at times. Especially at meal times. I'd see a few of them shovelling the food into patients' mouths and hear them say things like, 'If you don't eat this they're going to send you to the hospital and put a tube down your nose.'

Sometimes we even vent our frustrations on the furniture:

> I never told my husband this, but the reason the mirror is broken in the bathroom is because I slammed the bathroom door so hard the mirror broke. I told him I was trying to kill a wasp with a broom handle. I think he believed me. I was just so ashamed of myself for getting so angry that I'd actually started destroying the furniture.

Not all expressions of anger are healthy. Our angry outbursts can hurt other people. They can also make us feel guilty and ashamed of ourselves. But the emotion of anger itself is not always unhealthy or destructive. Anger can be a legitimate response to justifiable causes.

What makes us angry? Why? These are the two key questions.

Anger at God

'Whenever there is suffering, whether physical pain or mental anguish, man-at-his-best will do his best to help. But his powers are so limited. God's power, so they say, is unlimited. So why doesn't He *do* something?' wrote Hugh Silvester in the book *Arguing with God*.

C.S. Lewis, in *A Grief Observed*, also asked *Why?* when his wife was diagnosed with a fatal illness:

> What chokes every prayer and every hope is the memory of all the prayers [she] and I offered and all the false hopes we had. Not hopes raised merely by our own wishful thinking; hopes encouraged, even forced upon us, by false diagnoses, by X-ray photographs, by strange remissions, by one temporary recovery that

might have ranked as a miracle. Step by step we were 'led up the garden path.'

A bit earlier (three to four thousand years earlier) a man named Job also asked the *why* question as he sat on an ash heap, stricken by boils, grieving about his own physical suffering and the deaths of his ten children. In the book of Job, he bitterly cried out against the apparent injustice of God:

> I am tired of living. Listen to my bitter complaint.
> Don't condemn me, God. Tell me! What is the charge against me?
> Is it right for you to be so cruel? To despise what you yourself have made? And then to smile on the schemes of wicked men?

Today, people with Alzheimer's, and their carers, are still asking, 'Why?'

> My wife can't understand why everything happened to her the way it did. She said that if you believe in God, then things should be nice in life, even in old age. But things didn't turn out nice. They turned out terrible.

> When my mother got Alzheimer's I told God and the church goodbye. I figured if there was a God he could have prevented it. And if God didn't allow it to happen, maybe he caused it to happen. So who needed him.
> It has taken me years to get over my anger.

Why *doesn't* God do something about Alzheimer's disease? Why did he allow it to happen in the first place? There's one school of thought that says you shouldn't argue about the nature of God when a person is sick or dying. But when we are seriously or terminally ill or when someone we love is suffering or dying, that's the time we struggle most with these questions.

When things are going well for us (by *our* standards) we may rarely question God's goodness. It only becomes an issue when we're faced with a personal crisis.

My own struggles revolved as much around my own frustrated plans and desires as they did around my mother's disease and the devastating effects it had on both her and my father. For me, it wasn't so much an issue of the goodness of God in general as it was the goodness of God in particular. I suspect this is true for most of us.

Turning our thoughts away from ourselves can help us put our own situation in perspective. It can help us realize we're not alone in our grief. Others walk that road too, others who have concluded that even though they don't know all the answers, God has not abandoned them.

> I was angry at God for several years after my mother was diagnosed with Alzheimer's disease. Then I started going back to church. I decided to go for the sake of the kids, not so much because I'd got over my anger.
>
> The first day back, I saw a woman whose son had been killed in a plane crash and a woman in her thirties whose husband had died of a heart attack. I realized that though they'd been through all that suffering they still believed. I started crying. I cried through the whole service. That's what brought me back.

It is okay to be angry. It is not okay to stay angry for ever. Christopher Allison, in *Guilt, Anger, and God*, writes about this need to move beyond anger:

> It is strange that the cultural taboo against admitting

anger toward God has . . . made us regard it as shocking and something to be suppressed. The thought of expressing our anger toward God in worship is scandalous to many. Yet . . . the Psalms . . . are generously sprinkled with anger toward God for injustice on earth. Anger certainly is a major theme in the book of Job . . . Our sickness is our destructive anger. Our medicine is God's taking our anger. If we do not give it to him we are not healed of it.

Pain and suffering are not part of God's original plan. Disease and death were not part of the good world he created.

Those with Alzheimer's and those who care for them can cling to the promise that all things work together for good. Not that we'll necessarily be delivered from this present suffering, but that we have someone to walk through it with us. No matter how hotly our anger may burn.

Anger at Others

As Alzheimer's takes its toll on our emotions, we will be tempted to lash out at those around us, venting our anger at the expense of other people. To keep our cool, we may need to think about safety valves.

A safety valve releases excess pressure. Pressure cookers have them. When pressure inside becomes more than the pan can bear, an automatic valve on top releases the steam.

Carers need safety valves too. We need to know how to release our anger and frustration in *constructive* ways. We also may need to plan for the future and take preventive measures at the start to keep the pressure from building to explosive levels. Excessive pressure building up for the carer can result in explosions of uncontrolled anger.

Emergency measures for immediate situations may include some of the following:

- When tempted to verbally or even physically lash out at the person you care for, pull yourself together and count to ten. If necessary, walk away from the situation. If you need to vent your anger, pound a pillow, clean out a cupboard, scrub a floor, chop wood. Avoid throwing and kicking things. Caring is expensive enough without having to replace the furniture.

- Put yourself in your loved one's situation. Ask yourself, 'How would I like to be treated?'

The following paragraphs offer practical suggestions for defusing anger in less volatile situations.

Distraction is a useful tool we can use with Alzheimer's sufferers and ourselves. Distraction is anything that gives mental amusement, relaxation or diversion.

Laughing at a situation instead of getting angry or frustrated can be one way of lessening pressure and a means of distraction. You're laughing not so much at your relative, but at the situation. Laughter lets off steam. Your loved one may also appreciate a good laugh at times. I laugh with my mother a lot. I think it helps us both to remember that life was not meant to be gloom and doom; it's meant to be lived and enjoyed, even the difficult moments.

The apostle Paul had good advice for anxious and angry people: rejoice, be gentle, talk to God about your needs. All these things will bring peace of heart and peace of mind.

In addition, Paul encourages us to fill our minds with thoughts that are true, pure, lovely and praiseworthy. All of these thoughts make for peaceful meditation.

Martin Luther described this kind of meditation another way. He talked about letting our 'thoughts go for a walk.'

The scene before you may be one of utter chaos, but *you* don't have to be an internal wreck. When tempted to explode, turn your mind to some happy memory from the past or think about an anticipated event. Meditate on a psalm, a hymn, a quotation, or some beautiful aspect of the natural world.

When tempted to lash out at other loved ones, such as relatives who never call or visit, think about the possible reasons for their actions. Are they, too, having difficulty dealing with their loved one's illness? Do they need you to reach out to them and 'give them permission' to share their own feelings of grief? Talking to your relatives about your feelings may be the best thing you can do for you both. And if talking's not possible, forgive. Carrying a load of resentment inside will be only destructive.

If nursing-home staff or other health professionals do things or say things that anger us, we should let them know about it. Not by exploding in rage, but by talking to them about their attitude, their behaviour, the things we believe are negative responses.

Sometimes, because of our guilt, we may over-react and get angry about things that are normal for nursing-home life. At other times, our anger may be justified. Others may need help in viewing the situation through your eyes, the eyes of a carer. We all need to be sensitive to each other and to work together as a team. Honest, open communication can help make this possible.

There are also a number of preventive measures we can take to make the build-up of anger less of a problem. Because these are also good cures for depression, they are covered in the following chapter.

Anger at Alzheimer's

It's normal to be angry at Alzheimer's. It's a thief, a murderer, a destroyer of minds.

While ranting and raving at it won't do anyone any good, there are positive things we can do to help us feel more in command of this seemingly uncontrollable disease. We can channel our anger in practical ways by getting involved in the fight against Alzheimer's and other related dementias.

You may feel, as a carer, that you have neither the time nor the emotional or physical energy needed for involvement on any other level than an occasional support-group meeting. If you do have the energy, however, here are a few suggestions. Some can be done individually, others with a group:

- Help plan a seminar to educate other carers, health professionals and the general public about Alzheimer's. Your own support group could join with others in your region or plan with local hospitals, nursing colleges or community-service agencies.

- Order a box of supplies from the Alzheimer's Disease Society and set up a table to distribute them at community health fairs and town fêtes. Your office on ageing may also have information on Alzheimer's. Some other good resources for literature are found in Appendix D.

- Develop and distribute a newsletter for your area if none is available.

- Offer yourself as a speaker to nursing homes, hospitals, college classes on ageing and health, civic groups and churches. This could be a formal presentation, a simple question-and-answer session, a panel presentation.

- Ask a reporter from a local newspaper to write an article about Alzheimer's or submit one yourself. Raise public awareness of the disease and let people know what's available in the community.

- Support the Alzheimer's Association Disease Society. Many carers also encourage giving to the society at the time of the death of a loved one as a lasting memorial gift.

- Get involved politically. Be informed about local and national legislation related to caring issues and funding for Alzheimer's research. Write letters to your member of Parliament as well as to government ministers for health and social services. You can also let your views be known to your local councillor, the chairman of the local health authority, the chairman of the local social services and the Community Health Council for your area. Remember that the people who hold the purse strings at all levels of government need to hear from the people who know about the disease. The people most in the know are carers. Major issues to speak up on include that of financial support for carers. State benefits are currently inadequate in terms of paying for institutional care and carers' needs. Many people believe that they should be at least at the level of the state pension. You may wish to support Caring Costs, an organization which lobbies for an independent income for carers.

  Another vital issue concerns the availability and standard of care services, especially respite care. It must be recognized that regular short breaks are needed for carers, at least one half day per week. Alzheimer's needs also to be more widely acknowledged as a terminal illness so sufferers can qualify for the terminal illness level of Income Support. This would benefit patients, carers, and hospitals and homes which are often underfunded.

Most worthy causes became causes because someone got angry. A loved one was killed by a drunk driver or abducted from a schoolyard, died of cancer or suffered from Alzheimer's disease. The war against Alzheimer's is far from over. We all need to get involved in some battles and channel our anger in constructive ways.

CHAPTER FOURTEEN
Joy in the Mourning

'Be merciful to me, O Lord, for I am in distress; my eyes grow weak with sorrow, my soul and my body with grief. My life is consumed by anguish and my years by groaning; my strength fails because of my affliction, and my bones grow weak.' David, the author of Psalm 31, was depressed.

Depression is an emotion we all experience as carers. It can range from sadness to profound sorrow, sometimes accompanied by physical symptoms. It is triggered by many things.

Facing Depression

Depression can descend like a weight with the realization that we are no longer known by our loved one:

> They say it gets easier but I don't believe it. Each time I go to see my wife it gets harder for me. It's as if I were a total stranger. I hug her and kiss her and talk to her, but she doesn't know me. She doesn't know what's going on.

Depression can also be related to the death of expectations. Many who seem to have a bright and productive future suddenly see that future destroyed by a diagnosis:

> The real irony was that a week after my father was
> diagnosed he got a letter from a company he used to
> work for asking him if he'd consider being the execu-
> tive director.

Depression can be related to the fact that our relative is
not able to experience the joys of grandparenting:

> If I would start crying, my son would toddle upstairs,
> get some tissue, come sit on my lap, and pat me as if to
> say everything would be okay. The fact that my mother
> had this beautiful little grandchild who was comforting
> *me* because of *her* made my depression worse. I
> wanted so much for them to know each other, but I
> knew it could never happen.

Depression is often related to the anxiety, suffering and
depression our loved ones are experiencing. Their confusion
doesn't eliminate emotions like fear and frustration. They
also may have a sense of meaninglessness and have suicidal
thoughts that can be accompanied by actions:

> I've had people say to me, especially nurses, 'Don't
> worry about your father. You're suffering more than he
> is.'
> I cannot believe that. I see my father's emotions. I
> see his facial expressions and his behaviour. I say to
> myself, no one can tell me he's not feeling something. I
> don't believe that he's living in his own peaceful little
> world and that he doesn't know anything or anybody
> and he's not suffering. I do not believe that.
> I see signs of anxiety and frustration. I see the look
> on his face when he wants to say something and can't

get the words out.

I will never be convinced he's not suffering some.

———————

My wife used to have a tremendous will, not wanting to let anything get the best of her. Then, just before Christmas, she gave up.

———————

In the spring my husband tried to commit suicide. He got out one night when I was asleep. When I woke up, I called the police and we went searching. We finally found him up on the railroad tracks. There was a train coming. He said to the police, 'Leave me alone. Leave me alone. I want to die. I have a right to kill myself if I want to.'

Sometimes when we're depressed, the underlying problem is really our anger. One common definition of depression is 'anger turned inward.'

For months I was depressed. Months. My wife finally said to me, 'Honey, I don't think your problem is depression. I think you're just angry at what happened to your father.' She was right.

Searching for the Light

In his chapter on depression and loneliness in the book *Good Grief*, Granger Westberg likens depression to a dreadfully dark day when the sun is blacked out by clouds. People will always say, says Westberg, 'The sun isn't shining today.' But that's not true. The sun is shining, even when it appears not to be. Get on a plane, climb through the layer of clouds and eventually you'll see that the sun *is* shining. And someone will always make the remark, says Westberg, 'Too bad the people downstairs can't see this.'

The sunshine. The light moments. We need to look for those light moments in our loved ones' lives and not be afraid to enjoy them.

> We have our jokes, our light moments. We laugh at some of the things Dad does. He's very funny sometimes. Like the day he set off the fire alarm in the nursing home or the day he decided to take a walk outside. He wheeled another resident out the door too. The other man didn't want to go and was hollering 'No, no, no,' and carrying on. But Dad didn't care. It was a nice day for a trip.
>
> Dad always had this affectionate way of patting you on the bottom. He did it to me not too long ago, and I said to Mum, 'There, he's his old self. He did it again.'
>
> These little, light moments may last only a split second, but when they do appear they're good. They're very good.

Looking for the light moments is one way carers cope with depression. Another way is through *preventive* measures that may not eliminate depression for us and our loved ones, but can lighten the emotional load. They are also good ways to prevent the pressure from building up in our lives.

Maintaining Physical Fitness

If you spend half your day running around the neighbourhood in search of your relative or running up and down stairs ensuring his or her safety, you may be physically fit. Not all of us do this. Some Alzheimer's sufferers are confined to wheelchairs and lead very sedentary lives. So do some carers.

The benefits of exercise in relation to stress reduction are well documented. When our large muscles are exercised, our involuntary muscles also relax. Stress is reduced. We have more energy. We feel better all over.

- For me and several other carers I interviewed, swimming is a key to tension reduction. It helps ease depression and is a good way of keeping aerobically fit.

  When I became a full-time carer I thought my year-round swimming days might be over. The nearby lake was perfect for summer swimming, but the winter months loomed dark and dreary. Then I spoke with the director of our local swimming baths. 'Swim here,' he said. 'Your mum can come too.'

  Mum's 'going to the pool' consists of sitting downstairs in a comfortable chair next to the television and the front desk. I secure her with a restraint and usually put a little tag on the ties that reads, 'Please don't untie this. I'm a little confused. My daughter, Sharon, is in the pool.' She normally doesn't try to wander, but I'd rather be safe than sorry.

  Mum is very content to look through or rip pages out of magazines until I return. She also enjoys the children who run around and sometimes stop to talk to her. Any anger or depression I had going into the pool diminishes or disappears altogether after half an hour of laps.

  Some carers hire in-home help if they aren't able to take their relatives with them. Some have even learned to swim and have met new friends.

- If you're a runner, find a field or a track and take your relative with you. Let her or him sit and watch you huff and puff. A wheelchair ride around the block a few times can also be good exercise for you and a good outing for the person you care for. (Check with the Disabled Living

Foundation Information Service or surgical supplies shop for types of chairs best suited for this. Many are very sturdy and very portable as well. Sometimes this expense is at least partially reimbursable.)

- Golfing is another sport that many couples have engaged in in the dementia-free past. If so, don't think you have to give this up. Your relative may enjoy riding in a golf cart or, like my mother, sitting in the club house (restrained) in front of the window. (This, of course, only works when there are other people around.) If you golf during the week you can usually golf a few holes at a time and come back in to check on your loved one.

  Some people with Alzheimer's can continue to enjoy golf, tennis, bowling and other sports. They may no longer be able to keep score or play for as long as they used to, of course. But do continue to help them do the things they've always done for as long as they are able (if they can do them and not be frustrated by their diminished abilities).

- Maintain a balanced diet. This may seem obvious, but many carers (myself included) don't do it. A balanced diet for us includes food from the basic four food groups, the same as a balanced diet for those we care for. (See chapter eight.)

  In addition, the following recommendations should help us look better, feel better and be less fatigued and depressed:

  Eat food low in saturated fats and cholesterol (fruits, vegetables, cereals, pasta, low-fat dairy products, fish, poultry and lean meats).
  Limit salt intake by ignoring the saltcellar and avoiding highly salted, processed foods.

Cut calories if needed to attain and maintain your weight at recommended levels.

- Try to get adequate rest. The child's prayer that begins, 'Now I lay me down to sleep,' may be only wishful thinking for a lot of carers, but lack of sleep does play a part in depression. If you have sleepless nights and dreary days, consider hiring a helper for at least one of those nights so you can catch up.

Keeping Mentally and Emotionally Balanced

There are a number of things we can do to help us keep our own minds engaged and our emotions on an even keel.

- Develop your sense of humour. One carer made the statement, 'I think people that don't have a sense of humour are the people that are really in trouble emotionally.' Do appreciate those lighter moments in your loved one's life. Try reminiscing about the good, fun and funny times you've had together.

  Get acquainted with authors or poets who know the human condition and who can write about it with humour and wisdom, such as Garrison Keillor, Pam Ayres and Joyce Grenfell. Read articles that can touch your heart and lift your spirits.

  There's a proverb that says, 'Even in laughter the heart may ache.' We might also say that even in depression the heart may laugh. Without laughter, hearts can shrivel up and die.

- Maintain old hobbies and interests or develop new ones. Don't give up on the things you've enjoyed doing in the past—woodworking, reading, gardening, going to concerts, watching films. Incorporate your relative into your activities, if you can, or hire help for an hour or so each week (or find a volunteer) so you can get out and pursue your interests. That's a part of maintaining mental health. Both you and your loved one will be richer for it.

- A wheelchair can also be a worthwhile investment, not only for exercise but simply for going places. Even if your loved one is still able to walk well, wheelchairs can be useful for situations that require longer, more tiring walks.

  Over the past few years, with the aid of a wheelchair, I've been able to take my mother Christmas shopping, to the zoo, to museums and galleries, and even camping at a park equipped with caravans and nature trails designed for the disabled.

  Check with your local Department of Social Services or Borough Surveyors about acquiring a disabled vehicle badge for the windscreen of your car. Generally only those people who have permanent and substantial difficulty in walking are eligible for concessionary parking under the 'Orange Badge Scheme'. A doctor will have to sign a statement of need if the person does not already hold a mobility allowance.

- If music has been an important part of your loved one's life as well as your own, don't underestimate its value. Often the ability to play a musical instrument is still retained, though memory for other things is lost. Attend musical events together for as long as possible.

- Maintain relationships with other people or develop new relationships. You may find it impossible to go out much, but you can invite people in. Don't feel they wouldn't want to come. Most people enjoy being invited out to eat. Suggest they bring a dish to share if your budget is tight.

This may be a good way to get to know other carers, too, and provide an evening 'out' for all concerned.

- If depression is a chronic or severe problem over which you seem to have little control, you may need to seek professional assistance. There are many trained counsellors in private practice and local mental-health clinics available with counsellors on staff. Members of the clergy can also be good sources of support and are usually well acquainted with depression. Sometimes medication may be needed as well as counselling.

  Signs and symptoms of a more severe depression can include:

  generalized weakness/fatigue
  uncontrollable or frequent episodes of crying
  weight loss or, sometimes, weight gain
  low blood pressure
  headache or generalized aches and pains
  constipation
  sleep disturbances
  memory lapses or confusion
  symptoms of anxiety: tightness in the chest, stomach
      cramps, shaking, dizziness, a lump in the throat,
      sweating, diarrhoea, heart palpitations
  excessive drinking
  mood swings that range from euphoric to depressive
  negative self-concept; low self-esteem
  suicidal thoughts.

Seeking Spiritual Support

Spiritual support for both you and your relative can take many forms. One of the best support systems is a local church.

Church, of all places, should be a place where you can take your loved one even in times of bizarre behaviour. Church families that are sensitive to the needs of memory-impaired people and their carers will be able to come up with some creative ways to help you both enjoy various aspects of the worship experience, whether on a Sunday morning or at various times throughout the week. If you don't find this to be true, talk to the priest or vicar. You may have to make your needs known directly. You may also find you have to look around a bit for a church that meets your needs. Finding a good church can be a little like finding a good home-care worker. Sooner or later, with persistence and prayer, you'll find the right match.

One church I know of gives carers a break each Sunday by offering free home care. People in the church take turns looking after a woman's husband, who is memory impaired, so she can attend services. Another sponsors various carer support groups and offers training seminars on topics related to caring.

When I got over my own anger at God and was looking for a church, I knew for certain when I had found the perfect match. This knowledge hit me one Sunday when, in the middle of the pastor's sermon, the congregation began singing 'Home on the Range.'

The reason for the song was an elderly man named Hoppy, who suffered from dementia. Every Sunday the pastor's words would trigger something else in Hoppy's memory that related to a familiar song.

This Sunday the pastor was talking about going to our heavenly home. The mention of 'home' was all Hoppy needed to break into a chorus of 'Home on the Range.' The pastor just smiled and encouraged the congregation to join in. So we all stood and sang. This, I thought, is a group of people who are comfortable with people with dementia!

In *Good Grief*, Westberg writes about the church as a

place of healing, a place where our spirits can be lifted and where the depressed can truly see the sunshine through the clouds.

He writes: 'A congregation of religious people ought to live up to the well-known description of "the community of the concerned." If they are actually concerned about those who mourn, who feel lost from the world and from God, then they will earn the lasting gratitude of those who mourn.'

Finding Joy in the Wilderness

Depression has often been called 'a wilderness experience.' Many Alzheimer's sufferers know this to be true. They become lost in their own confusion and the tangled web of their minds. In the book *My Journey into Alzheimer's Disease*, Robert Davis, a Presbyterian minister diagnosed with Alzheimer's, writes about one aspect of his own wilderness experience:

> I go to church services to worship God, but I cannot sing. I cannot join in the readings or prayers because my mind cannot do two things at once. Singing and group readings take several processes going on at once to listen to the others and pace my reading in time with theirs. Such a simple thing. But impossible for me now.
>
> Suddenly I stand out in the worship service, silent and continually confused during the time of hymn singing. I feel that my fellow worshipers are looking at me askance, wondering why I do not join in. My new-found paranoia also sets in, making me wonder if they think by my silence I am showing disapproval of the hymn, the church, the musicians, or the people around me. This time of joy has been changed into a time of

frustration and anxiety.

Now I would like to come into the service late, after the singing of the first hymns or any responsive reading. However, out of propriety I do not. How I long to again sing my heart out and thus fully express my joy, but I cannot. The sorrow of this and this sense of loss fills me so much that often tears come to my eyes—tears that only compound my paranoia and my ever-present fears of what people are thinking.

As carers we also experience the empty, barren wilderness as we gradually lose our relative to a disease. As one carer asked, 'Where is the *essence* of my father?' The essence. Those indispensable, unique characteristics that make our loved one our loved one. Where are they? They're gradually lost with the progression of Alzheimer's disease, leaving us in a wilderness tinged with the memories of the past.

Elisabeth Elliot, in her book *Loneliness*, wrote the following: 'The wildernesses spoken of in the Bible were usually very barren places, but God can change that. He can make streams in the desert, springs in the valley, and furnish tables in the wilderness.'

Accepting our circumstances willingly can help turn our sorrow into joy.

Role-reversals

My mother used to call me Sharon. Then it became 'Honey,' the name she called me as a child. Pretty soon I became 'Mum' to her as her Alzheimer's progressed. And finally I became 'Gramma.'

For most people life is filled with roles. For carers, it's also filled with role-reversals:

Just when I thought the nest was empty, I find it filled

again. Not with grandchildren, but with my husband.

I see the role change with both my parents as I handle their affairs. I handle everything for them. I'm their mouthpiece, their spokesperson.

As soon as I moved back home, my mother saw me as the one in charge.

But I never looked on my parents as children. I just believe that now, in their senior years, they need more help. And I can help them.

I prayed for years, when I was away from home, for an opportunity to care for my parents in their old age if they needed it. I've accepted it and am thankful for it.

If we are not able to accept the role-reversal as part of a plan for our lives, we're never going to be able to experience true joy. The role of a carer can be a blessing or a curse, depending on our attitude. It can help us mature and blossom or it can cause us to wither away and die, emotionally and spiritually.

Yet we are not the only ones experiencing a role-reversal. Our loved ones are too. Robert Davis shares his own perceptions of the losses he experienced:

In my rational moments I am still me.

Alzheimer's disease is like a reverse ageing process. Having drunk from the fountain of youth one is caught in the time tunnel without a stopping place at the height of beauty and strength. Cruelly, it whips us back to the place of infancy. First the memories go, then perceptions, feelings, knowledge, and, in the last stage, our ability to talk and take care of our most basic human needs. Thrusting us headlong into the seventh stage of man, 'without teeth, without sight, without everything.'

At this stage, while I still have some control of thoughts and feelings, I must learn to take on the role of the infant in order to make use of whatever gifts are left to me.

Davis, unlike many people with Alzheimer's, was able to write about his feelings of loss. His book, written with his wife Betty, is a moving account of one man's journey into Alzheimer's, written by a man with a deep faith.

Perhaps the journey that takes me away from reality into the blackness of that place of the blank, emotionless, unmoving Alzheimer's stare is in reality a journey into the richest depths of God's love that few have experienced on earth. Who can know what goes on deep inside a person who is so withdrawn? At that time, I will be unable to give you a clue, but perhaps we can talk about it later in the timeless joy of heaven. On second thought, all these heartaches won't really matter over there, will they?

Part Four

SAYING GOODBYE

Death is not darkness.
It is turning down the lamp
when dawn has broken.
RABINDRANATH TAGORE

CHAPTER FIFTEEN

The Difficult Decisions

'There is a time for everything,' wrote the author of Ecclesiastes, 'and a season for every activity under heaven.'

Many will relinquish caring on their own for a season of residential care. For others, a season of caring at home will culminate in the death of a loved one. Neither change is easy; both bring a host of difficult decisions.

Knowing When to Give Up Caring at Home

It's time. Those two words are charged with a bushel full of conflicting emotions for carers who have finally made the decision to put their loved one in long-stay care. The decision never comes easily.

> My husband had been crying a lot. He kept saying, 'Help me, help me, help me,' over and over again. Nobody in the house was sleeping. Every day the furniture was turned upside down. He urinated in the middle of the kitchen. At weekends we just didn't bother with the house at all. People would come to visit and the chairs would be on top of the table. The couch was sometimes upside down. It was chaos.
>
> Then one day I was rung up at work. My husband was

at home, beating on the front door, crying and crying because he couldn't go out. One of the home-care helpers had called me, wondering what to do. A switch went on in my mind. I said to myself, 'It's time.'

The right time for long-term care is often related to the realization that we are no longer physically able to care for our loved one because of our own health problems.

I've heard people say 'I would never put my father or mother in a nursing home.' Well, I wouldn't have either if I could have handled him at home. But I couldn't. My mother couldn't. Physically we just couldn't handle it.

You have to be practical. You have to realize when you simply can't cope any more—physically or emotionally. When you can no longer give the people you love most the care they should have, that's when you have to decide.

———————

I had help for eight hours a day prior to putting my husband in a nursing home. That still wasn't enough. I was up all night, every night. And I'm eighty-eight years old. It got to the point where I knew it was either him or me, and I knew I wasn't ready for a nursing home yet.

Physical violence by our relative may be the last straw.

One morning my husband hit me on the shoulder. He'd threatened me a good number of times, but he'd never actually done it before. It didn't really hurt, but it scared me.

Just then the phone rang. It was my daughter. I was

crying as I told her what had happened. She immediately called the social-service worker who was already providing some home-care help for us.

The social worker came to see me that afternoon. That was a Monday. On Thursday my husband was admitted to the nursing home, one fairly close to our home.

I was glad he was going to that particular home. I'd visited it once before and liked it the best of any of them. That made the decision a little easier.

For others, safety may be the trigger issue—safety for our loved one and other family members.

Daddy kept falling. We tried to prevent it, but the only way was to keep him restrained in a chair, and he fought that so. The other alternative was to sedate him, but then it was impossible for me to physically handle him. So we finally decided that, for his sake and mine, the nursing home was best.

The day my mother set the waste-paper basket on fire in the bedroom was the day we decided to do something. She just wasn't safe any more.

So circumstances make us decide. Yet we still have to deal with our tangled emotions. And the predominant emotion is guilt.

Often, guilt surfaces because of others' attitudes:

There are so many people who think you put your parents in a nursing home because you want to get rid of them, that you don't want to be bothered, that you no longer care, that you don't appreciate what they did for you. They don't realize those are not the reasons at all.

Fortunately, the initial guilt is often followed by relief; based on our situation, we have made the best decision for all concerned.

Don't be surprised, however, if ambivalent feelings remain:

> Mum still feels guilty at times, but she knows Dad is getting good care.
>
> Mum really does worry about him. She prays for him every day. And I take her to see him once a week. She's prepared, if anything happens, to accept it.
>
> We might be distressed if Dad were anywhere else but the home he's in. It's good, it's clean and it's close. They're kind to him there. The doctor comes in every Friday and goes over his records and visits with him. The doctor's on call if there's a problem.
>
> All things considered, it's the best we could ask for.

> There was a lot of guilt. The nursing home was the last place I ever wanted Daddy to go.
>
> When I went to visit him, I'd sit in the car and pray for strength to go in and go through all the conflicting emotions I knew I'd have. I'd pray that I could act cheerful.
>
> That first week I just wanted to pack Daddy up and take him home. I even thought of quitting my job to take care of him. But, even while I was thinking about it, I knew I couldn't. I knew it wasn't the best. For me. For my family. For Daddy.

I still feel guilty whenever I visit my wife.

The other night I went to see her and she hugged me and kissed me and seemed to know who I was. I cried. I couldn't help it.

But when she is not good and doesn't know me and doesn't pay any attention to me, I'm glad she's where she is.

So I'm up. And I'm down.

———————————

I do feel guilty because I don't get to the nursing home as often as I used to. In the beginning I saw my father every other day. But then I suddenly realized there are other things that need to be taken care of.

My mother, who's still at home, has needs too. Lots of them. I'm running her house too. She can live alone but she can't do her own cooking. I cook at home and make up frozen dinners for her.

I'm simply not always able to get up, get out, and go see my father every day.

We may wonder, 'Did I make the right decision?' But the day will come when we know certainly the answer is yes.

In the beginning it was hard. Dad always wanted to come home with us. When it was time for us to leave, we'd say to the nurses, 'Please get Dad's attention.' And the nurses would try to distract him while we crept out.

Then one day when we were getting ready to go, Dad turned to us and said, 'You know, girls, this isn't a bad place. I rather like it. I think I'll buy it.'

All of a sudden, our guilt about institutionalization was gone.

In the midst of this difficult decision making, some carers long for the good old days, an era when life was simple and families stayed together through thick and thin. Nancy Mace and Peter Rabins, in *The 36-Hour Day*, put the good old days in perspective:

> We tend to think of the 'good old days' as a time when families took care of their elderly at home. In fact, in the past not many people lived long enough for their families to be faced with the burden of caring for a person with a demential illness. The people who did become old and sick were in their fifties and sixties and the sons and daughters who cared for them were considerably younger than you may be when your parent needs care in his seventies and eighties. Today many 'children' of an ailing parent are themselves in their sixties or seventies.

Times have changed. For today's families, the first goal is to support a loved one in whatever environment best meets his or her needs.

The second goal is to rid ourselves of the guilt that comes when nursing-home placement is necessary. It may help to remember that up to sixty per cent of nursing-home beds are filled with people who suffer from Alzheimer's disease or a related dementia. We are not alone.

What Are the Options?

There are really a number of options available for caring away from home.

The Residential Care Home. Residential homes are designed for people who don't require regular medical or nursing care but who cannot live alone because of age, poor health or a chronic disability. Not all homes will accept people with Alzheimer's, and some may take only a certain quota. On the other hand, more homes are now being opened exclusively for dementia sufferers. However, unless they are among the few homes 'dual registered' for both residential and nursing care, they may not be able to keep patients when they become totally disabled and need more intensive nursing care. In practice, because residents are still able to receive the usual community nursing services and the care of their doctor, they may be able to remain in residential care without being transferred.

A social worker may help you obtain a place for your relative in a council-run ('Part III') home. If you ask in advance, it may be possible for your loved one to have a trial stay or perhaps to visit on a day basis.

The same is true of profit-making private residential homes and the non-profit making voluntary homes. Size and type of accommodation and standards of care vary tremendously and it is impossible to make generalizations. Check that the home is registered with the local authority and inspected regularly (a legal requirement). Talk with other carers and with groups like Age Concern if you are in any doubt. Many people prefer residential care because of the homely atmosphere and personal attention offered.

Hospital Care. Many Alzheimer's sufferers are placed in the geriatric wards of general hospitals or in psychiatric hospitals. They may first spend time in an assessment ward after a doctor's examination and referral. Care in hospital may be on a long-term basis or for occasional periods, providing respite for the carers. National Health Service hospital care is free, but your relative's National Insurance Pension will be reduced after the first eight weeks as a contribution to care.

Dementia Units. Some hospitals and nursing homes have special-care units for people with dementia. These are usually secured wards that allow people to freely wander in a supervised environment. Your local group of the Alzheimer's Disease Society may be a good resource for specific information.

Nursing Homes. There are various types of nursing homes. Very few are run by the NHS; most are privately run, and some are run by voluntary organizations. Nursing care is provided by qualified staff twenty-four hours a day and a qualified nurse or doctor will be in charge.

Quality varies from home to home and has little to do with a home's profit or nonprofit status. From my own experience, I have found that quality depends on the training and attitudes of the personnel.

Looking for a Nursing or Residential Home

There are many things to consider when looking for a suitable home. The following points may help make things easier.

- Talk to other carers who have placed relatives with Alzheimer's in homes. How did they choose that particular home? Are they happy with it?

- Seek out nurses, social workers or others in your community who work with the elderly (specifically with Alzheimer's sufferers). Ask what's available in the area.

- Keep your own limitations and the concerns of family in mind. For instance, there may be an excellent home several hours away that has a special unit for people with

Alzheimer's. Is this an option? Would visitation by family and friends still be possible?

● Meet with your relative's GP. It's good to have a doctor involved early in the planning process, for information and support. Also, a doctor's referral will usually be needed for admission to a nursing home.

Unfortunately, many carers shop for a nursing home as they shop for Christmas presents. At the last minute.

This is unwise. Plan ahead. This will enable you to choose the home best suited to your relative's personality and needs. Don't wait for a crisis and then expect a bed to be available. Chances are, it won't.

Reasons for advance planning include the following:

Waiting lists. Some homes have them, others don't. Even if you're unsure about placement, it's wise to fill out an application at a number of homes. (You can always say no if you are called and are not ready to place. Just ask the home to call you again in the future.) Sometimes many months go by before a bed is available. With hospitals discharging patients quicker and sicker, some homes are more likely to admit directly from the hospital itself.

Some homes limit the number of people they will admit with a demential illness. In this case, it's essential that you be placed on a waiting list.

Legal loose ends. There's always a need to explore legal issues related to nursing-home placement. It takes time to tie up loose ends. Don't shortchange yourself.

Additional Criteria

The Good Care Homes Guide, published by Longmans in association with Care Home Consultants and in consultation with Help the Aged, selects and grades private residential homes and nursing homes in England and Wales. The Alzheimer's Disease Society also has an information sheet entitled *What to Look for in Residential Care*, available through its London office. This is well worth obtaining and reading.

In addition to using a guide or checklist, evaluate a nursing home or any other similar facility with your own common sense and common *senses*.

Visit several facilities. Planned visits with the nursing-home social workers and/or nursing-home administrators are essential, but you may also want to arrive unexpectedly, too. Talk with some of the residents and their families. Observe the residents involved in activities both social and health related. Watch the nursing-home staff at work. Pay attention to first impressions and to what your senses are telling you.

What do you *feel?* Does the place feel like a home or an institution? Even in very large homes, caring, compassionate, non-institutional attitudes will show—if the staff have them.

What do you *see?* The best homes combine good nursing care with a homelike atmosphere. Are individual rooms cheerful, with pictures on the wall and mementoes from home? Are the majority of residents out of bed, dressed in street clothes and well groomed? Do most appear alert? *Alert* does not necessarily mean 'oriented.' It has more to do with wakefulness. If the majority of residents are not alert, it may be a sign of inappropriate medication.

Do the nursing assistants (the people doing most of the hands-on care) look frenzied and frazzled or do they appear relatively calm and relaxed? Ask about the aide-to-resident ratio; you'll want to know if the home is adequately staffed.

What do you *hear*? Pay attention to what people are saying and their tone of voice. Do the staff talk to the residents? What do they talk about? Do they speak to them with dignity and respect?

Don't be unduly upset if you hear residents shout or scream at times. Bath and shower times are prime occasions for this; confused residents may resent this intrusion or be frightened.

What do you *smell*? It's not possible to have a completely odour-free environment in a nursing home. You may note the smell of urine or stool coming from a room or two as you walk down the corridor. This should be an exception rather than the rule. If there is a pervasive odour of urine or some other unpleasant smell, ask why. You should also see housekeeping staff mopping and damp dusting.

Ask the nursing director what kind of training staff receive. It is also worth trying to find out what philosophy they have on the issues of patients' rights, the problems of ageing, safety, and so on.

How Do I Pay the Bills?

One of the first questions a nursing home will ask the family of a prospective resident is, Who will pay the bill? Nursing homes usually aren't cheap. But their cost covers nutritious meals, your relative's share of the rent and utilities, and medical care that involves many trained personnel.

Paying for all of those benefits can be handled in a variety of ways, including the following:

Private funds. Some families are able to pay for nursing home care privately, though not necessarily for ever. Costs will vary and may increase annually.

Spouses, children and other responsible parties will need to consult with a lawyer about their own financial liability and issues of concern. For example, are you legally and financially responsible for a parent in a nursing home? For all or part of their care? Talk with the nursing-home social worker, but don't sign anything until you've also checked with your own financial adviser.

Benefits. With the high cost of nursing care, it is vital to be aware of any benefits to which you or your relative is entitled. These include invalidity benefit (payable to a person incapable of work, up until retirement age) and the retirement pension. Widow's benefits include an initial lump sum, the widowed mother's allowance, and widow's pension (for those with no dependent children). Varying criteria apply.

Income Support and/or housing benefit may also be claimed by those in residential or nursing homes, to help with fees.

No benefits are paid automatically and a written claim must be made, in some cases with medical evidence. Claim forms are available from local post offices, Department of Social Security Offices and Citizens Advice Centres, and specialist advice can be obtained from the Alzheimer's Disease Society or Age Concern.

Insurance and pensions. Private health insurance and certain life insurance and pension plans may also cover some nursing-home costs. Some plans are excellent, while others pay negligible amounts for custodial-type care. Talk directly with your insurance agent or a company representative about available benefits.

Veteran benefits. If your loved one is a war veteran or the spouse of a veteran, enquire about benefits. It is also worth finding out about any veterans' nursing homes in your area.

Making That Difficult Decision

As you weigh the pros and cons of placement, consider the following issues and questions. Your responses should help you make a wise and appropriate decision based on your loved one's needs and the needs of your family.

Health. Can you continue to care for your loved one at home without jeopardizing your own mental, emotional and physical health? What about the health of other family members? Is the care you're able to provide keeping your relative as healthy as possible—or is ill health increasing in frequency, duration or intensity?

Safety. Can you continue to provide a safe environment, or are accidents increasingly beyond your control? Is the safety of the rest of the family at risk if your relative remains at home?

Support. Do you have enough support from family, friends and community services to handle increasing care needs? Is the help you need (or will need) affordable as well as available?

Placing my own mother in a nursing home was not an easy decision for me. I was one of those people who had always told myself, 'I'll never do it.' But then, one day, I did, just like other caregivers have done. Health, safety, and support were all factors in making the decision. It seemed that Mum and I were spending more and more time on the floor; she was no longer able to walk as the Alzheimer's progressed into the final stages, and transfers from chair to bed or wheelchair to car were becoming increasingly difficult. Safety for both of us was an issue coupled with dwindling finances and a decision I had made to move to another city to continue my education. Mum's unexpected trip to the hospital for a condition unrelated to her Alzheimer's was the trigger event that convinced me that 'now was the time'. Friends and relatives were supportive, realizing better than I that home care was not really providing the best for her, no matter how well I thought I was coping.

Continuing to Care

You can still care for a loved one in practical ways after he or she moves to a nursing home or hospital. Relinquishment does not mean abandonment. In fact, a good home will welcome any support you can offer. This includes visits as well as helpful hints—drawn from your years of experience—about caring for your relative.

- People who are confused do better in familiar surroundings. Suggest arranging the furniture as it was at home, if this is possible. Some homes will even allow you to bring in familiar furniture. Also bring pictures, photographs and, of course, your relative's favourite clothes.

- Be with your loved one on the day of admission. You won't necessarily need to stay all day, but several hours will be helpful for the initial transition. Take someone with you for support—another family member or a best friend. Don't assume an Alzheimer's sufferer won't adjust. Sometimes they settle in immediately; if they no longer recognize familiar faces, everyone may be family to them.

- Before admission or on the day of admission the social

worker will want to know more about your relative's background. This is called 'taking a social history.' As a nurse, I find social histories to be vitally important. The history might include the type of work your loved one used to do, places of employment, special hobbies and interests, information about children and grandchildren (including names and addresses), religious affiliation and involvement, languages spoken, and so on. Unfortunately, on some charts the information is very sparse, either because there was no family to give it or because families felt the information was too personal.

The activities department of the home can use this information to plan a programme suited to your relative's needs. For example, if your loved one was very active in church, provisions can be made for attending worship services and special religious services in the home. Other activities might include social hours, film showings, bingo, baking. A person with Alzheimer's may not be able to participate actively in these activities but may enjoy socializing in a group.

A social history also can be helpful for the nursing assistants caring for your loved one. Knowing something about your loved one's interests and occupation can provide a point of contact for conversation or provide the carers with something to talk about.

Anne Evans and John Smith exemplify the value of a detailed social history. Anne Evans was a resident who had been very depressed. I attended one of the care conferences when the staff talked about possible reasons for her depression and suggested ways to cheer her up. Leafing through her social history, I noticed that she had been an avid golfer. I went home that night, wrapped up a new package of golf balls and brought it in the next day. Anne and I unwrapped the package together. This small action didn't cure her depression, but it brightened her day and provided a point of contact. She enjoys talking about her past interest, and that has opened the door for discussing other concerns as well.

John Smith was a patient who had been comatose for over a year. A nursing assistant told me, 'I always turn his radio to classical music when I take care of him. One of his relatives told me he played the violin and was in an orchestra when he was younger.' That information wasn't part of Mr. Smith's social history. I added a note to the chart and we put a sign on the radio about keeping it tuned to a particular station.

These pieces of helpful information can easily be forgotten in the busyness of admission procedures. Feel free, though, to pass them along (preferably in writing) at any time, so they can be shared with staff members and benefit your loved one.

• Continued visiting is important. Some people visit daily, others weekly, others less frequently. There is no right or wrong schedule. Feel your way into a visiting schedule that meets the needs of everyone involved.

Visiting doesn't always have to be in the home. Plan to take your relative out: go to a restaurant, have a picnic in the park, go shopping or attend church. Going back to his or her previous home may or may not be an option to consider. Some people easily adjust to this; others want to stay home once they get there. Some people with Alzheimer's experience increased stress related to outings and home visits and may actually be better off remaining in the home; don't feel guilty if this is the case, even on holidays that are normally family occasions. The nursing home staff will be honest with you if you ask them about how your loved one readjusts to the home routine after a home visit.

When you visit, use the time to care for your loved one in

practical ways. Give a manicure, go for a walk or a wheel-chair ride, assist with feeding at mealtime. Actually doing something physical may help you feel better about the visit.

Continuing-Care Issues

Once your relative settles in, concerns will continue to arise. Talk to the charge nurse, social worker or director of nursing about any problems. Remember, though, that some things will be done much differently than they were at home. For example, your loved one may need to wear a restraint when in bed or sitting up to protect against falling or injuring other residents. If you have any questions about the type or quality of care given, talk with the people in charge. Let your concerns be known.

- Take advantage of planned activities that enhance staff and family relationships. This can be a less stressful time to get to know the staff more personally. Nursing homes truly are extended families in many ways. These types of activities, when everyone is really enjoying each other's company, can help you see the home or hospital as a caring community of friends.

- Inevitably, questions arise concerning terminal care. If a loved one suddenly stopped breathing, what should be done? Should he or she be resuscitated?

  In some facilities all staff are trained in CPR (cardiopulmonary resuscitation) and would be expected to try to revive any resident suffering a cardiac or respiratory arrest. In other homes staff would immediately call an ambulance. The ambulance team might then attempt to resuscitate.

  It is wise to discuss your feelings about resuscitation of

a terminally ill relative with the staff and possibly the social worker of the nursing home. Planning ahead can make things easier for you and your loved one.

- Finally, stay in tune with your feelings. Be involved in a support group. Some nursing homes have support groups that regularly meet in the home. Ask about them.

Guilt, anger and depression do not automatically disappear the day you walk through the nursing-home door or the day you walk out and leave your loved one behind. But we can deal with all these emotions the same way we dealt with them when our relatives were home, with the understanding that what we're experiencing is normal. We *will* survive.

The Post-mortem and After

My grandfather said, 'No post-mortem. Your grandmother's been through enough hurt already. We don't need to do that to her.'

_____

I've made plans for my father's brain tissue to be donated. As a matter of fact, I have a post-mortem file.

When I left for a holiday recently I told a friend, 'Here's the file. If anything happens to Dad, get the file to my brother. He'll have to act immediately.'

I have the materials filed both in the nursing home and at the hospital where Dad's doctor practices, so they'll know this is what we want.

It's a very difficult thing to plan. Just the thought of what they'll have to do hurts me terribly. But if it can help future victims—if it can help future generations of our own family—it will be worth the tears.

_____

At the time we didn't understand the need for research. Now we wish we'd had the autopsy done.

When I'm alone, bored, and the weather's nasty, I think about Mum's death and the post-mortem. I know it had to be done.

There was the chance that they would find something in her brain that would give them a clue as to what really goes wrong. And I know my mother would have said, 'Do it, if it's going to help someone else.'

Requesting a post-mortem examination (or autopsy) of the brain, and arranging the donation of brain tissue, is a final step that many carers decide to take, for a number of good reasons.

Post-mortems conclusively confirm or deny the presence of Alzheimer's disease. During an autopsy, the pathologist microscopically examines sections of the brain. If Alzheimer's was present, there will be plaques and tangles, the disease's main characteristics.

If Alzheimer's was the cause of the dementia, treatment for symptomatic relatives may be possible. Family members could then take advantage of experimental-drug research and medical advances if diagnosed early.

Families will want also to know if plaques and tangles are absent. For people worried about the disease's genetics possibilities, such news can offer relief.

The only other test that can conclusively confirm or deny Alzheimer's is a brain biopsy, performed while the patient is alive. These are rarely done. (Biopsies require both extensive samples and the subject's informed consent.)

Post-mortems contribute to Alzheimer's research. Studying the living brain is difficult. Unlike other major organs, the brain is not easily probed. It's encased in a bony 'safe' designed to protect it from infection and trauma.

The brain also has the added protection of a special membrane called the blood-brain barrier, which prevents undesirable chemicals from entering the brain. This protective sheath makes it equally difficult to withdraw any foreign chemicals from living brain tissue, chemicals that might give clues to Alzheimer's cause.

Alzheimer's is a uniquely human disease that affects our thoughts, emotions, personalities and wills. Animal models, useful for research in many other diseases, are unsuitable for researching a disease of the mind.

Post-mortems help generate funding for research. Funding for research for any disease is based largely on its prevalence. In the case of Alzheimer's, it's especially important that accurate statistics are gathered.

These factors highlight the importance of brain-tissue research. A cure is unlikely unless a cause is discovered, and no cause will be discovered without continuing exploration into the abnormalities of autopsied human brain cells.

Consenting to a Post-mortem

Without an autopsy, doctors are usually reluctant to cite Alzheimer's disease as the cause of death. This reluctance does a disservice to you, to the memory of your loved one and to future generations. It will only be eliminated if family members consent to autopsies.

The decision to have a post-mortem done, or to donate brain tissue, should not be left to the emotion-laden days surrounding the death of a loved one. A sudden, unexpected death might even eliminate the opportunity for an autopsy because of the necessary requirements. Foresight and planning are essential.

A great deal of information, guidance and support is needed before a decision for a post-mortem can be made. Help is available from a number of sources.

- Start with your local support group. Ask others in the group if they have gone through this process. Have a speaker on the subject come to a meeting and discuss the regulations that apply to your community.

- Think through the reasons for a post-mortem and weigh the pros and cons. You may have religious objections. Talk to your pastor, priest or rabbi if this is a concern for you.

  You may feel that your loved one's body will be desecrated or treated with disrespect. Rest assured that a brain autopsy causes no disfigurement to a person's face or body. There is no reason why, following an autopsy, you cannot have an open-casket viewing or funeral.

- Discuss the decision with family members. If there is a surviving spouse, the ultimate decision rests with him or her. Still, it is good to agree as a family—and all family members will have an opinion on the subject, coloured by their emotions and knowledge of what's involved.

- Send for the information sheet on Brain Tissue Donations from the Alzheimer's Disease Society. As well as suggestions for practical arrangements, this includes a list of research centres which would be grateful for the donation of post-mortem material for further study.

Making Medical Arrangements

Talk with your relative's doctor and staff of the nursing home to find out what arrangements will be needed for an autopsy.

Make sure that you speak to your relative's doctor and/or staff of the nursing home to find out what arrangements will be needed for a brain autopsy. You may need to make special arrangements in case your loved one should die at a weekend or on holiday, and there may be a time limit involved.

If you have decided on brain tissue donation, contact the nearest research centre in good time, for the necessary information. Forms will need to be filled in and plans made with the local pathologist. In some cases there will be costs for transportation to the research centre.

Remember also that the funeral director must be involved and aware of your wishes. The body should not be embalmed before the brain is removed.

Knowing the Truth

Several months after an autopsy, you or your doctor should receive a written, detailed explanation of the results from the neuropathologist. This will include a diagnosis based on both large-scale and microscopic findings.

Consenting to a post-mortem is never a painless decision for anyone who is a carer. After all the suffering our loved one has experienced, we may feel he or she is entitled to rest in peace. But if we see the autopsy or tissue donation as an aid to research and the ultimate diagnostic test for a disease that, someday, may be arrested, prevented and cured, it becomes a pain that offers promise.

For us, our loved ones and our families, the battle may soon be over. For millions of others, it has only just begun. The information gained from our relative's post-mortem may be the vital link in the chain that will one day reveal the true cause of this devastating disease known as Alzheimer's.

CHAPTER SIXTEEN

Blowing Out the Candle

Muriel sat at the kitchen table. The wick in the paraffin lamp flared, casting a warm glow over the chilled room. The storm had abated but the electricity was still out. Muriel sat, stared at the flame, and thought about her mother's death several days earlier.

Her mother's death had been a lot like that flickering wick. A lot like the dimly burning candle that sat on the mantel in the dining room.

Death had not come easily for Ruth. Neither had life. She had always worked so hard. Worked hard raising three children. Worked hard on the farm with her husband. And when she developed Alzheimer's, Ruth worked incredibly hard, for many years, to cover it up.

Then Ruth had died hard—labouring to breathe, to stay alive, to keep the fire of life burning.

Muriel remembered that some of her friends, children of parents with Alzheimer's, said death was a relief. It was a release from years of suffering. Muriel wasn't so sure. It didn't seem like that for her mother. What was death really like? What would it be like for her? Was it a foe to be fought or a friend to be welcomed?

Muriel lowered the wick in the paraffin lamp and watched as the smoke curled around inside the glass globe. She walked over to the candle on the fireplace mantel. One blow. Two. A third finally snuffed the flame.

Just like Mum, thought Muriel. Just like most of us— working hard to keep our candle burning.

Caring for the Dying

For some loved ones, death will come quietly, quickly. For others it will come only with more struggles, more suffering. The way of death is not something we can explain or understand. We can merely wait, prepare and pray that we can make it a little easier for our loved ones and ourselves.

When the nursing home called me about a change in my mother's condition, it was the week before Easter. I made the four-hour trip out to see her and planned to go with her to the hospital for a series of tests related to gastrointestinal bleeding she had developed. But just prior to her scheduled tests, Mum's condition deteriorated and it was soon apparent to all concerned that the primary concern was now related to her breathing.

I was faced with a decision. My mother's doctor gave me the options: acute hospital care or comfort care at the nursing home with a staff well equipped to keep my mother as pain-free and comfortable as possible. I chose the latter course of action and spent the next three days (and most of the evenings and nights) sitting at her bedside, holding her hand, and assisting the nurses and aides with her personal care. When death came, it was not without a struggle, for both of us; but it came as I would have hoped it would. Mum was not alone. It was clearly evident from the tears of the nursing assistants that I was not the only 'family member' who had loved her.

The following suggestions, written prior to my mother's nursing home experience and ultimate death, are ones I would still recommend, with a few additions based on my own, more personal, experience.

Caring for someone approaching the final days of life is not very different from caring for any other very ill person. Keeping your relative comfortably positioned, clean, dry and as pain free as possible are goals.

The following suggestions will make your loved one more comfortable if confined to a bed and in need of total care.

- Keep the room well aired and well lighted. Good ventilation makes breathing easier and provides a more pleasant environment for you to work in. A dark room can be a frightening place for someone who is dying, especially someone with Alzheimer's.

- Because of poor circulation, your relative may feel cold. This will be especially noticeable in the hands and feet. Lightweight blankets and comforters will help.

- Skin care is vitally important as poor circulation and inadequate nutrition take their toll on the body's ability to nourish cells. Turn the person frequently, at least every two hours. Give soothing back massage. Pay special attention to the skin over any bony prominences like the hips, bottom of the spine, heels, elbows, shoulders and even the back of the head and the ears. Consider obtaining a water, air or foam mattress for the bed to prevent skin breakdown.

- Heels and elbows can be padded and wrapped with gauze if your relative thrashes against side rails. Sheepskin and foam booties are also available.

- Position extra pillows to increase comfort and decrease pressure on legs and arms.

- Bowel and bladder control will diminish even more until there is total incontinence. Keep your loved one as clean and dry as possible. A laundry service, if available, will help greatly.

  A catheter, which may be inserted by a district nurse with a doctor's order, may help remove urine from the bladder. This can easily be maintained at home, provided the person is relatively still and doesn't pull it out.

- Keeping your loved one hydrated and nourished will become increasingly difficult. The ability to swallow may eventually be lost altogether. In the meantime, provide favourite foods that are high in calories.

  When swallowing becomes more difficult, offer custard, yogurt, pureed fruits, ice cream. Sometimes milk products and citrus fruit juices will increase mucous production and cause problems. If this is the case, switch to non-dairy products and juices such as apple and grape.

  Ice chips may be welcome if sucking can be done without danger of choking. When swallowing becomes more of a problem, moisten a face-cloth in ice water and let your loved one suck on it.

- Good mouth care is essential. Your relative will probably breathe through the mouth, and the jaw will sag. The mouth can become very dry and uncomfortable as a result. Frequent liquids can help, but also consider purchasing some mouth swabs. Use them often.

- Placing a very light layer of petroleum jelly on lips and around nasal passages may help prevent cracking.

- If the person is bothered by an excessive amount of mucous build-up in the mouth, rent a suction machine.

- A sitting or semi-sitting position is best for eating and can help prevent choking. (Renting or borrowing an adjustable hospital bed will make this more practical.)

One investment which you can make at any time during your loved one's illness is a good nurse's-aide or nursing-assistant manual. Such manuals offer hundreds of additional tips on how to feed, position, bathe, toilet and otherwise meet the physical needs of people who are ill. In some areas, a Terminal Care Service may be avail-able to assist carers in nursing those who are dying at home.

Should terminal care prove overwhelming for you, consider getting assistance through a hospital or hospice. The latter features professional carers and volunteers who emphasize pain control and meeting the physical, emotional and spiritual needs of patient and carer, in as natural an environment as possible. Some agencies offer sliding fee scales based on ability to pay.

Emotional Support

'What is it about death that makes you afraid?' I once asked an elderly woman in a nursing home.

'The dying part,' she replied.

'But what about the dying part?' I asked, hoping she'd be more specific.

'The part about dying alone,' she said.

We can provide emotional support for loved ones simply by being with them. We can hold their hands, offer back massage and remind them that we love them. We can pray for them, and we can assure them they won't be abandoned. They are not alone.

That is all our loved ones really ask of us. To sit and wait with them for the door of death to open.

Spiritual Support

I once led weekly Bible studies in a nursing home with a small group of Alzheimer's sufferers.

Our favourite passage, and one we read frequently, was Psalm 23. It is a psalm about death. It is also a psalm about life—eternal life. It recognizes that death does not have to be a lonely experience. There is someone to walk through the valley of the shadow of death with us. Remind your loved one of this; remind yourself.

Brightly Burning Wicks

A number of years before my mother's death I broke her walking stick. It happened the morning I was late for work because the helper I had hired was late. 'My car broke down,' she said on the phone. 'I'll be there when I can.'

Frustration. I was supposed to be covering for a sick co-worker at the office. I had to get there as soon as possible.

My mother wasn't helping at all. When I tried to get her out of bed, she resisted. When I finally got her on her feet, she decided to sit down on the floor. That's when she began striking my legs with her stick. She didn't hit me hard, but I lost control. I grabbed the stick and banged it against the floor. The cane, old and fragile, snapped in two. It lay broken on the floor beside my mother.

I felt shame and horror. My first thought was 'What if that had been my mother?' Would anger or frustration ever make me treat her like that stick?

Mum brought me back to the present. She was still sitting on the floor. But now she was laughing. I sat down beside her, put my arms around her and laughed too. I laughed until I cried.

That night I read this verse from the book of Isaiah: 'A bruised reed he will not break, and a dimly burning wick he

242

will not quench.' That struck a nerve. At times, I felt like a bruised reed, bruised and battered in the battle against Alzheimer's.

My mother was a bruised reed too, a fragile person incapable of caring for herself or understanding what was happening. A person who needed to be cared for gently—with love, laughter and, occasionally, tears.

But the verse in Isaiah holds a promise. Neither of us will be broken. Neither of us has to walk through life alone, despite the suffering and confusion. God has promised to hold our hands. He will also *stay* my hand and give me patience with my mother and myself.

Later, I hauled the broken stick out of the rubbish and put it in the linen cupboard. It is still there, a reminder for me to be gentle with my mother and with others whose lives are flickering in the darkness.

It reminds me, too, that we are not alone.

Appendix A

Checklist for Evaluating a Nursing Home

1   Does the home have a current licence from the
    local health authority?

2   Does the home provide special services, such
    as a specific diet or therapy, which the patient
    needs?

PHYSICAL CONSIDERATIONS

3   **Locations**
    a   pleasing to the patient?
    b   convenient to a doctor?
    c   convenient for frequent visits?

4   **Accident prevention**
    a   well-lighted inside?
    b   free of hazards underfoot?
    c   handrails in hallways and grab bars in bathrooms?

5 **Fire safety**
   a meets fire regulations?
   b exits clearly marked and unobstructed?
   c written emergency-evacuation plan?
   d frequent fire drills?
   e exit doors not locked on the inside?
   f stairways enclosed and doors to stairways kept closed?

6 **Bedrooms**
   a open onto a hall?
   b windows?
   c no more than four beds per room?
   d easy access to each bed?
   e nurse-call bell by each bed?
   f fresh drinking water available?
   g at least one comfortable chair per person?
   h reading lights?
   i wardrobe and drawers?
   j room for a wheelchair to manoeuvre?
   k care used in selecting room-mates?

7 **Cleanliness**
   a generally clean, even though it may have a lived-in look?
   b free of unpleasant odours?
   c incontinent patients given prompt attention?

8 **Vestibule**
   a welcoming atmosphere?
   b if also a lounge, is it being used by residents?
   c furniture attractive and comfortable?
   d plants and flowers?
   e certificates and licences on display?

9 **Hallways**
   a large enough for two wheelchairs to pass with ease?
   b handrailing on the sides?

10 **Dining room**
   a attractive and inviting?
   b comfortable chairs and tables?
   c easy to move around in?
   d tables convenient for those in wheelchairs?
   e food tasty and attractively served?
   f meals match the posted menu?
   g those needing help receiving it?

11 **Kitchen**
   a food preparation, dishwashing and rubbish areas separated?
   b food needing refrigeration not standing on counters?
   c kitchen help observe hygiene rules?

12 **Activity Rooms**
   a rooms available for patients' activities?
   b equipment (such as games, easels, wool)?
   c residents using equipment?

13 **Isolation Room**
   a at least one bed and bathroom available for patients with contagious illness?

14 **Toilet Facilities**
   a convenient to bedrooms?
   b easy for a wheelchair patient to use?
   c washbasin?
   d nurse-call bell?

e handrails on or near toilets?
f bath and showers with non-slip surfaces?

15 Grounds
a residents can get fresh air?
b ramps to help handicapped?

SERVICES

16 Medical
a doctor available in emergency?
b personal doctor allowed?
c regular medical attention assured?
d thorough physical immediately before or upon admission?
e medical records and plan of care kept?
f patient involved in developing plans for treatment?
g other medical services (dentists, opticians, physiotherapists and so on) available regularly?

17 Hospital
a arrangements with nearby hospital for transfer if necessary?

18 Nursing Services
a Registered nurse responsible for nursing staff in a registered nursing home?
b Licensed practical nurse on duty day and night in a registered nursing home?
c trained nurses' aides and orderlies on duty in homes providing some nursing care?

19 Rehabilitation
a specialists in various therapies available when
   needed?

20 Activities
a individual patient preferences observed?
b group and individual activities?
c residents encouraged but not forced to
   participate?
d outside trips for those who can go?
e volunteers from the community work with
   patients?

21 Religious Observance
a arrangements made for patient to worship
   as desired?
b religious observances a matter of choice?

22 Social Services
a social worker available to help residents and
   families?

23 Food
a planned menus for patients on special diets?
b variety from meal to meal?
c meals served at normal times?
d plenty of time for each meal?
e snacks?
f food delivered to patients' rooms when necessary?
g help with eating given if needed?

ATTITUDES AND ATMOSPHERE

24   General atmosphere friendly and supportive?

25   Residents retain human rights?
   a   may participate in planning treatment?
   b   medical records are held confidential?
   c   can veto experimental research?
   d   have freedom and privacy to attend to personal needs?
   e   married couples may share a room?
   f   all have opportunities to socialize?
   g   may manage own finances if capable?
   h   may decorate their own bedrooms?
   i   may wear their own clothes?
   j   may communicate with anyone without censorship?
   k   are not transferred or discharged arbitrarily?

26   Administrators and staff available to discuss problems?
   a   patients and relatives discuss complaints without fear of reprisal?
   b   staff responds to calls quickly and courteously?

27   Residents appear alert unless very ill?

28   Residents who are out of bed are wearing day clothes?

29   Visiting hours accommodate residents and relatives?

30   Civil-rights regulations observed?

31   Visitors and volunteers pleased with home?

Appendix B

Other Causes of Dementia

There are a number of chronic disease processes that can produce dementia-like symptoms, and persons with these symptoms can be misdiagnosed as having Alzheimer's. In certain cases, symptoms of these other diseases can be controlled with medication and the disease process slowed. Known risk factors for some chronic disease processes may be modified.

I. Vascular Dementias

Multi-infarct dementia (MID). MID is one type of vascular dementia and the second most common cause of chronic irreversible dementia in older adults. Its cause is multiple strokes or infarcts in the brain related to an atherosclerotic process that narrows arteries feeding brain cells; when brain cells are not fed enough oxygen and nutrients because blood flow is cut off, they die. (This process is similar to what happens when someone has a heart attack and blood flow to cells in cardiac tissue is compromised.) MID is often a corollary to untreated diabetes or hypertension.

Symptoms associated with MID may seem to appear suddenly, though multiple-stroke or mini-stroke activity has been occurring over a period of time. Persons with MID may experience periods of confusion and then periods called plateaus where there seems to be no perceptible change in memory or behaviour; this process differs from the slow, steady, global decline associated with Alzheimer's. Persons with MID may exhibit specific local or focal neurological impairment related to specific areas or brain involvement, for example, slurred speech or muscle weakness in an arm and/or leg.

To complicate diagnosis, Alzheimer's disease and MID can coexist, and frequently do, in what is called a 'mixed-dementia' that may account for fifteen to twenty percent of all existing chronic dementias.

Differentiating Alzheimer's from MID through various neuro-imaging techniques is of great importance. Though multi-infarct dementia is not considered reversible, further stroke activity and associated dementia may be preventable as many of the risk factors for MID are known and controllable (for example, hypertension, diabetes, and vascular disease). Surgical, dietary, lifestyle, and pharmacological interventions may be indicated.

Binswanger's disease is another vascular dementia associated with persistent, severe hypertension. Risk factors also include diabetes, cardiovascular disease, and recurrent hypotension. Advanced arteriosclerosis in the medullary arteries occurs with pathologic changes in the frontal subcortical white matter of the brain.

Symptoms of Binswanger's disease include difficulty swallowing (dysphagia) and difficulty articulating words (dysarthria). Difficulty walking, frequent falls, and urinary incontinence may also occur. Binswanger's is also plateau-like in progression. Control of associated risk factors may help slow or halt disease progression. Neuro-imaging techniques are used to diagnose Binswanger's.

II. Prion-Related Dementia

Creutzfeldt-Jakob disease (CJD). CJD is a rare form of dementia believed to be caused by a transmissible prion protein. Though symptoms are similar to Alzheimer's, including memory impairment, behaviour changes, and compromised coordination, Creutzfeldt-Jakob disease has a rapid progression, with death occurring within a year of diagnosis.

Symptoms may also include sudden jerking movements (myoclonus), an exaggerated startle reflex, and epileptic seizures. This disease can be diagnosed by brain autopsy following death due to unique pathological changes in brain tissue; while living, there may be abnormal EEG readings.

III. Neurotransmitter Abnormalities

Parkinson's disease is caused by the absence of dopamine, a neurotransmitter that controls muscle activity. People with Parkinson's may also experience dementia in the late stages of this illness. In the early stages of Parkinson's, slowed or delayed thinking processes may be evident but, unlike the Alzheimer's sufferer, a person with Parkinson's, given time, will be able to remember and reason even though speech may be slower than normal. These two diseases are often confused in both early and late stages.

To confuse matters more, persons with Parkinson's may actually develop Alzheimer's, and persons with Alzheimer's may exhibit symptoms more typically characteristic of Parkinson's, for example, joint stiffness, slow movement (bradykinesia), difficulty walking or initiating movement, and sometimes complete immobility. One feature unique to Parkinson's disease and usually absent in Alzheimer's is tremors or mild to severe shaking of the hands and head.

Medication can help alleviate symptoms associated with

Parkinson's, specifically the medication levodopa or L-dopa. Antidepressants are also often ordered to combat depression frequently associated with the disease.

IV. Hereditary Dementias

Huntington's disease or Huntington's Chorea. This is a hereditary disorder involving early stage cognitive changes, memory impairment, and involuntary movements (chorea) of the face and upper extremities. Depression, hallucinations, and paranoia may also occur early in the disease and progression may be a slow deterioration.

A genetic marker identified on chromosome 4 has been linked to the Huntington's gene. Pathological changes in the brain include marked atrophy, extensive nerve cell loss, and a decrease in white matter.

Various medications may help control abnormal muscle movements, though they often lead to rigidity as a side effect. Tricyclic antidepressants are often used to combat depression.

V. Motor Neuron Abnormalities

Amyotrophic lateral sclerosis (ALS). ALS is often called "Lou Gehrig's disease" after a famous baseball player who was one of its victims. It is characterized by progressive muscle wasting and weakness, involuntary contractions of the face, tongue atrophy and difficulty speaking, and spasticity. ALS may be due to an excess of the chemical glutamate that is responsible for relaying messages between motor neurons. Too much glutamate destroys nerve cells in the brain and spinal column.

Mental and memory changes are generally not associated with this disease, unlike many other neural degenerative diseases. ALS is commonly seen in people in their late thirties and forties.

VI. White-Matter Abnormalities

Multiple-sclerosis (MS). MS is a progressive, degenerative disease with myelin sheath and conduction pathway involvement of the central nervous system. White fibre tracts connecting white matter and neurons in the brain and spinal column are usually affected. Causative explanations include viral, immunologic, and genetic factors. CT scanning may show increased density in the white matter and MS plaques. MRI and PET scanning may also be used.

As MS progresses, memory loss, impaired judgment, and and inability to problem solve and perform calculations may occur. Earlier symptoms include generalized muscle weakness, fatigue tremors when performing activities, numbness and tingling sensations, visual disturbances, dizziness and ringing in the ears, and disturbances with bowel and bladder function.

Because symptoms are often vague and can mimic other diseases, MS often goes undiagnosed and cognitive symptoms can easily be misinterpreted for Alzheimer's disease. MS typically occurs in the twenty- to forty-year-old age range.

VII. Other Degenerative Disorders

Pick's disease (PKD). A rarer form of dementia, PKD often manifests itself in disturbances of mood and a progressive inability to speak (aphasia) that may render a person totally mute.

Disinhibitions of a sexual nature and inappropriate social behaviours and loss of social awareness are more indicative of Pick's than of traditional Alzheimer's dementia; memory loss is not as profound as in Alzheimer's disease. Behavioural disturbances may occur later in the disease that may include hyperorality or bulimia and visual agnosia or inability to interpret visual images. PKD initially affects people in their fifties and sixties.

Like Alzheimer's , Pick's disease can best be diagnosed by brain autopsy. Plaques and tangles will be present as well as 'Pick bodies' in cerebral cortex, basal ganglia, and some brainstem structures. On a CT scan, severe atrophy may be present, especially in the temporal and frontal areas of the brain.

Appendix C

Medications and Research

Research and the development of new experimental drugs is ongoing and ever-changing. The following is a brief summary of the latest in Alzheimer's research in the past ten years.

I. Free Radicals and Antioxidant Therapy

Researchers have long studied the beta amyloid protein that accumulates in the brains of persons with Alzheimer's disease. Recent research suggests that this protein also produces free radicals, or molecules, with odd numbers of electrons that in turn are known to cause cell damage or cell death. Earlier research has shown that some antioxidants, for example, vitamin E, protect cells from naturally occurring free-radical damage.

Clinical trials have included the experimental medication *deprenyl*, believed to block free-radical damage, and vitamin E that may serve to neutralize the toxic effects of free radicals. Carers should not give their loved ones excess doses of over-the-counter vitamin E. Excess doses of any vitamin are highly toxic.

II The Genetic Question

In 1987 researchers discovered evidence for a gene(s) on chromosome 21 related to Alzheimer's disease specifically in some families with early-onset familial Alzheimer's disease (FAD). FAD occurs in one to ten per cent of all persons with Alzheimer's disease and has been known to occur in persons in their thirties. Chromosome 21 is the same chromosome associated with the occurrence of Down syndrome abnormalities in the brain that occur in persons with Down syndrome by age forty are similar to those occurring in the Alzheimer's victim, including the characteristic plaques and tangles. Also in 1987, the gene that contains the code for the amyloid precursor protein (APP) was found on chromosome 21. APP is related to beta amyloid protein and senile plaque formation.

In 1992 the APP gene on chromosome 14 was found to contain a mutation(s) associated with early-onset familial Alzheimer's disease cases that affected persons in their forties.

In 1993 chromosome 19 was found to have a genetic mutation more than three times as common in persons with late-onset FAD and sporadic AD (no 'known' relatives had Alzheimer's disease) than in persons without Alzheimer's disease. This gene is called apolipoprotein E (ApoE). ApoE appears to be the first biological risk factor for late-onset Alzheimer's (other than age itself).

The study of the ApoE gene is one of the most promising avenues of research. In the future there may be ways to reduce a person's risk of developing Alzheimer's, for example, by manipulating metabolism to postpone Alzheimer's, according to Duke University researchers.

III. Environmental Factors

Though to date the only established known risk factors for Alzheimer's disease are age, family history, and genetic predisposition, researchers believe some factor(s) in the environment may also play a part in the development of the disease. The study of various metals in the environment such as aluminium, mercury, and zinc is ongoing. To date the research has yielded mixed results.

Chelation therapy is sometimes advertized in popular self-help magazines as a means of ridding the body of excess aluminium or zinc. But the side effects, including hypotension, vomiting, anaemia, irregular heartbeat, congestive heart failure, and kidney failure, far outweigh the proposed benefits. Carers should seek advice from the Alzheimer's Disease Society or a reputable medical centre before subjecting their loved one to any treatment.

Another environmental area of exploration is related to electromagnetic fields (EMFs) from power lines and other electrical equipment. A study reported in the American Journal of Epidemiology in September 1995 found increased likelihood of dementia in persons exposed to frequent and high levels of EMFs; this research needs to be replicated before conclusions can be reached about possible links between Alzheimer's and EMFs.

Long-term exposure to pesticides is also considered to be a possible risk factor for dementia and is under investigation.

IV. Acetylcholine Research and Related Medications

The experimental drug THA (Tacrine) was first tested in 1986. The drug was designed to inhibit the breakdown of acetylcholine in the brain, a substance known to be depleted in the brains of people with Alzheimer's and believed to be associated with memory function. It has more recently been approved by the US Food and Drugs Administration as the first drug released for the treatment of mild to moderate Alzheimer's. One side effect is liver toxicity, common to other experimental drugs. The jury is still out as to its effectiveness.

ENA 713 is another drug currently being used on an experimental basis. It inhibits the enzyme responsible for acetylcholine breakdown.

V. Mitochondria Research

Mitochondria are slender microscopic filaments. They are considered the source of energy for cells and are involved in protein synthesis and lipid or fat metabolism. Acetyl-l-carnitine naturally occurs in human cells and effects the proper functioning of mitochondria. The drug Alcar is currently being tested on an experimental basis at a number of sites in the US in people of ages forty-five to sixty-five.

VI. Vascular Dementia Treatment

Propentofylline (HWA 285) is a drug that improves blood flow and the metabolism of energy in the brain. It has been used experimentally in some research centres across the US.

Appendix D

Useful Organizations

Age Concern England
Astral House
1268 London Road
London SW16 4ER
Tel: 0181-679 8000

Age Concern Ireland
3 Lower Crescent
Belfast BT7 1NR
Tel: (01232) 245729

Age Concern Scotland
113 Rose Street
Edinburgh EH2 3DT
Tel: 0131 220 3345

Age Concern Wales
4th Floor
1 Cathedral Road
Cardiff
South Glamorgan CF1 9FD
Tel: (01222) 371566

Alzheimer's Disease Society
Head Office
2nd Floor
Gordon House
Greencoat Place
London SW1P 1PH
Tel: 0171-306 0606

Association of Community Health
Councils for England and Wales
30 Drayton Park
London N5 1PB
Tel: 0171-609 8405

Attendance Allowance Unit, DSS
Warbreck House
Warbreck Hill
Blackpool FY2 0YE
Tel: (0345) 123456

British Red Cross Society
Local Office

Carers National Association
Ruth Pitter House
20-25 Glasshouse Yard
London EC1A 4JS
Tel: 0171-490 8818

Caring Costs
Ruth Pitter House
20-25 Glasshouse Yard
London EC1A 4JS
Tel: 0171-490 8818

Citizens Advice Bureau
Local Office

Counsel and Care for the Elderly
Twyman House
16 Bonny Street
London NW1 9PG
Tel: 0171-485 1566

Crossroads Care Attendant Schemes
10 Regent Place
Rugby
Warwickshire CV21 2PN
Tel: (01788) 573653

Dial UK (The National Association of
Disablement Information and Advice Lines)
Park Lodge
St Catherine's Hospital
Tickhill Road
Doncaster
South Yorkshire DN4 8QN
Tel: (01302) 310123

Disability Alliance
Universal House
88-94 Wentworth Street
London E1 7SA
Tel: 0171-247 8776

Disability Living Allowance Unit, DSS
Warbreck House
Warbreck Hill
Blackpool FY2 0YE
Tel: (0345) 123456

Disabled Living Foundation
380-384 Harrow Road
London W9 2HU
Tel: 0171-289 6111

Elderly Accommodation Counsel (EAC)
46A Chiswick High Road
London W4 1SZ
Tel: 0181-995 8320

Grace Link
35 Walnut Tree Close
Guildford
Surrey GU1 4UL
Tel: (01483) 304354

Help The Aged
St James Walk
London EC1R 0BE
Tel: 0171-253 0253

Holiday Care Service
2nd Floor
Imperial Buildings
Victoria Road
Horley
Surrey RH6 7PZ
Tel: (01293) 774535

Invalid Care Allowance Unit, DSS
Palatine House
Lancaster Road
Preston
Lancashire PR1 1HB
Tel: (01772) 899508

Law Centres Federation
Duchess House
18-19 Warren Street
London W1P 5DB
Tel: 0171-387 8570

Legal information:
The Public Trust Office
Protection Division
Stewart House
24 Kingsway
London WC2B 6JX
Tel: 0171-269 7000

MIND (National Association for Mental Health)
Granta House
15-19 Broadway
Stratford
London E15 4BQ
Tel: 0181-519 2122

National Association of Citizens Advice Bureaux
115-123 Pentonville Road
London N1 9LZ
Tel: 0171-833 2181

Registered Nursing Home Association
Calthorpe House
Hapley Road
Edgebaston
Birmingham B16 8QY
Tel: 0121 454 2511

St John's Ambulance Brigade
Local branches in England and Wales

St Andrew's Ambulance Brigade
Local branches Scotland

Scottish Council of Disability
Princess House
5 Shandwick Place
Edinburgh EH2 4RG
Tel: 0131 229 8632

Winslow Press Catalogue
Winslow Press
Telford Road
Bicester
Oxfordshire OX6 0TS
Tel: (01869) 244733

Youth Access
1A Taylor's Yard
67 Alderbrook Road
London SW12 8AD
Tel: 0181-772 9900

ALZHEIMER'S ONLINE: INTERNET INFORMATION

1. The Alzheimer's Association's Home Page internet address is: http://www.alz.org/

The Home Page provides information about Alzheimer's disease, including caregiving strategies, research updates, and education and support opportunities. Also listed is contact information for more than 200 chapters nationwide. You can access it 24 hours a day. The Alzheimer's Home Page will also direct you to other organizations or freenets. An example of a freenet service available through internet is the opportunity to 'talk' with other caregivers in your own local area.

2. The Alzheimer's Disease Education and Referral Center (ADEAR) of the National Institute on Aging (NIA) also has a web site offering publications and research news. Web site is: http://www.alzheimers.org/adear

Available through ADEAR is a Progress Report, highlighting all the latest Alzheimer's research. Information specialists will also answer your questions about Alzheimer's disease.

Call the ADEAR Center at 001 (800) 438-4380, or contact them by E-mail at: adear@alzheimers.org

3. The Down Syndrome World-Wide Web site is: www.nas.com/downsyn/

INDEX

INDEX